Dr. Gaynor's
CANCER
Prevention
Program

Dr. Gaynor's

CANCER

Prevention
Program

Mitchell L. Gaynor, M.D.

AND

Jerry Hickey, R.Ph.

WITH

William Fryer

𝆎

KENSINGTON BOOKS
http://www.kensingtonbooks.com

KENSINGTON BOOKS are published by

Kensington Publishing Corp.
850 Third Avenue
New York, NY 10022

Library of Congress Card Catalog Number: 98-066229
ISBN 1-57566-382-1

First Printing: January, 1999
10 9 8 7 6 5 4 3 2

Printed in the United States of America

Text design by Stanley S. Drate/Folio Graphics Co. Inc.

Authors' Note

All dosages suggested in the sections labeled Pharmacist's Corner are for adults only.

If you have questions on the herbs, supplements, or medical foods referred to in this book, you can contact Dr. Gaynor or Jerry Hickey at the following e-mail address:

hickeychemists@jerryhickey.com
or
www.jerryhickey.com

Disclaimer

The nutritional information in this book is not a substitute for professional medical care. Because everyone is different, a physician must diagnose individual conditions and supervise treatment of all health problems. If you are undergoing medical treatment, consult your physician before taking any supplement. We urge you to seek the best medical resources available to help you make informed decisions.

The patients featured in this book have consented to the use of their clinical vignettes. To protect their privacy, we have changed their names, transposed events, and altered identifying characteristics.

Dr. Gaynor's Acknowledgments

My intention in writing *Dr. Gaynor's Cancer Prevention Program* has been to foster a dialogue between scientists, doctors, nutritionists, and patients. This dialogue gained momentum with the creation of the Anne Fisher Nutrition Center at the Strang Cancer Prevention Center and continued with my collaboration with Jerry Hickey, R.Ph., in writing this book. Through my work and research with doctors and scientists at Cornell University Medical Center, Beth Israel Medical Center and Rockefeller University, I have been fortunate to exchange ideas with experts whose pioneering studies you are about to read. I would like to express my gratitude to all the colleagues who supported and influenced me during the three-year process of writing this book: Andrew Dannenberg, M.D., Michael Osborne, M.D., Dr. Leon Bradlow, Dr. Devra Lee Davis, Dr. Frank Lipman, Dr. George Kessler, Dr. Anthony Antonacci, Dr. Jeff Friedman, Dr. George Gorham, Dr. Larry Dossey, Dr. Kenneth Kafka, Dr. Wayne Isom, Dr. Muzen Kamen and Dr. Carl McDougal.

I would like to also offer special thanks to William Fryer and Ron Young whose creative input and editorial suggestions contributed so much to this book.

Jerry Hickey's Acknowledgments

I'd like to thank Carl Germano, R.D., and Jay Lombard, D.O., for alerting Kensington Publishing Corp. to our existence. A special thanks goes to Lee Heiman for recognizing the importance attached to this work, and for his energy and dedication in making this book a reality.

I want to thank Allan Graubard and Paul Dinas for their editing expertise and the time spent with us poring over the documents.

This book is a user-friendly guide for decreasing the odds of ever having cancer. It is based on decades of expertise. I want to thank my research assistant Anne Marie Meehan for helping to collate, review, and critique the volumes of scientific research needed to write this book.

A special thanks to my friend and partner, Rob Martin, for always being there and offering both spiritual and intellectual support, and for his tireless commitment to the cause of cancer prevention.

I want to acknowledge and thank my wife Jo Ann for capably managing our business and allowing me time for both researching and writing. Thank you, and I love you.

And a very special thanks to my boys Alex and Matt, who at such a young age understood the importance of this book and allowed me to take precious time and attention away from them.

Thanks to Bill Fryer for helping to meld Mitch and my own writing styles.

To my patients
—Mitchell L. Gaynor

For my wife, Jo Ann, and my two boys,
Alexander and Matthew, with love.
—Jerry Hickey

Contents

Introduction

With the help of this book, you will most probably be able to protect yourself from cancer for the full length of a long life. The things you choose to eat are certainly capable of providing such protection. In my family, from my one- and seven-year-old sons to me, my wife, and my 74-year-old father, we're fully confident of that and adhere to a phytonutrient cancer prevention diet.

Why do we do so? My mother died of breast cancer when I was nine years old, and I don't want to have that experience repeated for any of us or for any of you, my patients and readers.

The greatest cancer breakthroughs of our time have occurred over the past decade without fanfare. These are not breakthroughs in treatment—treatment remains extremely difficult—but breakthroughs in prevention. They are steps as specific to stopping cancer before it starts as wearing a seat belt is to lowering your risk of a fatal automobile accident.

These great prevention breakthroughs are the reason for this book. They are exciting to forward-looking physicians throughout America. They are becoming the basis for a whole new physical understanding of what we are. They vastly increase the likelihood that most of us can live long and healthy lives in reasonable harmony with our own nature.

Going from the beginning to the end of a long life without ever encountering cancer is the way things ought to be for the vast majority of people. Half a million Americans shouldn't be dying of this painful, humiliating, and debilitating plague each year. Definitively and defiantly, no! Yet—wait a moment—that's how many are dying. It's a death rate exceeded only by those for heart disease and stroke.

There are real reasons why cancer continues to loom so large in the mortality statistics, why medicine seems stuck in a cancer rut, why the war on cancer seems the quietest losing war we've every fought. The truth, which most cancer specialists only recognize reluctantly, is this: what we've been doing up till now offers much room for improvement. Yes, we do our best in the struggle to cure cancer. Yet those efforts cannot equal the effects of doing our best to *prevent* it.

The preventive approaches discussed in this book are highly effective and well tested, and an emphasis on them goes back to the founding mission statement of the Strang Cancer Prevention Center in New York. By *prevention,* we don't mean things you should avoid. Truthfully, we won't be spending an awful lot of time discussing the *don'ts* of cancer prevention. If you haven't heard that you shouldn't be smoking, for instance, you probably won't be reading this book.

What the two of us—one, an experienced oncologist and the other, a noted nutrition pharmacist—want to tell you about are the vast range of *do's* that can change the way your body functions and feels. This is the world of phytonutrients, substances that have been specifically designed by nature to protect us. We now have the ability to draw on all the foods from all the culinary cultures of the world that protect against cancer. We are learning that such substances as soy and garlic, among a host of others, are not accidentally central to the cooking experiences of diverse civilizations.

Because of all that we have learned, we can now construct designer foods, isolate particular nutrients when needed, and combine diverse nutrients to make a genuine attack on the chain of events that cause malignancies in one of every three Americans at some point in their lifetime. We, the authors of this book, are at home in a whole new world of prevention, and we think it is essential that you become at home there, too.

I, Mitchell Gaynor, am currently director of medical oncology at the Strang Cancer Prevention Center in New York and assistant clinical professor of medicine at the New York Presbyterian Hospital-Cornell Medical Center in New York.

I, Gerard (Jerry) Hickey, am a leading nutrition pharmacist and chairman of the Society of Natural Pharmacy who owns two licensed pharmacies in Manhattan and the Hickey Nutrition Center on Long Island. I am cohost of Heathline, a nutrition talk show that airs Monday through Friday on WEVD radio.

For purposes of clarity and economy, we have written this book in the first person. It will be evident when one of us is speaking from his own particular experiences.

We believe that we are part of a movement to create a richer, broader, more successful form of medicine, but to create it, we need your cooperation. For most people, prevention will not come from something written on a prescription pad. You, the reader, and your friends and relatives and neighbors will need to arm yourselves against adversity. Nothing unpleasant there. Your defensive armor will be soft, tasty edibles intelligently laid out on a bed of common sense.

Eating well and feeling healthy, you will be able—in a dangerously unhealthy world—to avoid an atrociously undesirable illness. There is a world beyond cancer and the fear it evokes; it is beyond comparison better than the world we live in now.

—Mitchell Gaynor, M.D.
Jerry Hickey, R.Ph.

The precautionary principle*

We must act on facts, and on the most accurate interpretation of them, using the best scientific information. That does not mean we must sit back until we have 100% evidence about everything. Where the state of the health of the people is at stake, the risks can be so high and the costs of corrective action so great, that prevention is better than cure. We must analyze the possible benefits and costs of action and inaction. Where there are significant risks of damage to the public health, we should be prepared to take action to diminish those risks even when the scientific knowledge is not conclusive, if the balance of likely costs and benefits justifies it.

Source: Richard Horton, Editor-in-chief, Lancet.
*Modified from a 1990 UK Department of the Environment definition.
Lancet, Vol. 352. No. 9124, 25 July, 1998

CHAPTER 1

PHYTONUTRIENTS AGAINST CANCER

*After the ship has been sunk, everyone
knows how she might have been saved.*

—ITALIAN PROVERB

W hy shouldn't we make a major effort to *prevent* cancer?

As I go through life tussling with the day-to-day decisions of cancer therapy, I am teased and tormented by that question.

My work as a cancer specialist ensures that each day, I see great suffering. I make fierce efforts to alleviate it. I reassure my patients, I work with them, I comfort them, and when I can, I cure them. I struggle—as does every oncologist I know—to find effective treatments for a disease that is tenacious and proverbially hard to manage.

But always, that question tugs at me: "Couldn't all this have been avoided? Can't we prevent many of these tragedies from happening in the first place?"

We can. In fact, you can—and you should.

It is foolish to wait for this secretive and slowly nurtured disease to arrive before responding to its challenge. Too many people are the casualties of such an approach; and mainstream medicine's treatments, as everyone knows, are far from universally victorious. It is you who must make the effort at cancer *prevention.* I hope you'll have a committed and nutritionally alert physician beside you as you do, because that will certainly help, but even if you don't, you can make a major lifestyle decision that most probably will alter your medical future.

The prevention of cancer is not exactly a mystery anymore. For the most part, we know what causes cancer. We also know that our most faithful defenders are to be found in copious abundance in the plant kingdom that surrounds us, the green world without which our lives would be inconceivable. Scientists now call those defenders phytonutrients. *Phyto* is Greek for *plant;* therefore, phytonutrients are *plant* nutrients. These phytonutrients are so remarkably powerful when taken in sufficient number that they have

3

the capacity to free us from the fear of cancer by dramatically lowering our probability of ever contracting it.

Hundreds of fruits, herbs, and vegetables possess this protective power. Everything from that daily apple to the olive oil I hope you'll learn to cook with is important here. Even the miso soup you most likely haven't been eating at your local Japanese restaurant can work for you. In fact, almost all fruits and vegetables have at least a few protective natural chemicals on the outer surface of their skins or hidden within their pulp or meat.

Does this whole phytonutrient theory sound too simple? Perhaps you're saying, "Dr. Gaynor, everyone I know eats fruits and vegetables, yet some of these people get cancer. What gives?"

The truth is that quantity is every bit as important as quality. This applies in the world of protection, just as it does in the world of risk taking. Someone who smokes three packs of cigarettes a day is far more likely to get lung cancer than is someone who smokes just one. In precisely the same way, a person who consumes six or seven servings of cancer preventive powerhouse nutrients daily is far better protected than a person who eats one fruit at lunch and one helping of vegetables at dinner and says, "I've eaten my fruits and vegetables. Thank heavens I'm safe."

If I ate the way most people in this country eat, I'd be terrified for my life.

DR. GAYNOR'S STORY

Let me tell you how I came to practice the medicine I do and write the book you're reading.

I grew up in a small town in Texas. After obtaining my medical degree at the University of Texas Southwestern Medical Center in Dallas, I came to New York to do my residency. Then I went to Rockefeller University as part of my hematology–oncology research fellowship to study the immune system. The doctors I worked with there—including Jeff Friedman, M.D., who later became famous for discovering the obesity gene in mice—had a profound and growing knowledge of the effects of nutrients on genes, including cancer genes. It was very clear that these nutrient–gene interactions had a critical role in the immune system and in disease prevention.

I was flabbergasted. It would almost be fair to say that in medical school and during my hospital residency, nutrition was never stressed for any reason. Clearly, however; some of the best scientists in the country knew better. Working with them, I discovered that there were thousands of published scientific reports detailing the effects of foods and nutritional supplements on cancer. These reports, though read by research scientists, had never been translated into actual medical care.

I asked myself how I would bridge that gap. That was when opportunity knocked. Hearing of my interest and knowing of my training in oncology, Drs. Andrew Dannenberg, Michael Osborne, and Leon Bradlow at the Strang Cancer Prevention Center suggested I come work with them. The Strang Center was becoming more and more involved with nutrition medicine and was combining it with the conventional treatments for cancer—surgery, chemotherapy, and radiation. This was the combination I wanted to use in treating patients, so in 1994, I started working at Strang. In 1996, I was introduced to Jerry Hickey and we began devising nutritional combinations for cancer prevention.

JERRY HICKEY'S STORY

When I was a little boy growing up in Ireland, we were healthy and robust and so was almost everyone we knew. Taking perscription medication was not common. Herbs, cod liver oil, and other nutritional and traditional infusions of nature's own chemicals were our medicines.

When I came to America and later went to pharmacy school, the emphasis was very different. It was clear that the only important things we were going to learn about were prescription drugs. The focus on chemotherapy in cancer care was total. I can remember once suggesting the possible uses of nutrition and herbology in pharmacy class. Everyone laughed.

When I graduated in 1978, I started to look into nutrition on my own. I had seen the serious side effects that were associated with so many prescription drugs. I was hoping to find other answers for at least a few of life's common problems. By the time I owned my own pharmacy, I knew that nutrition could do a good deal more than that. In 1996, when Mitch Gaynor and I met, we resolved to look for nutritional combinations that would have major effects in preventing cancer. One result of combining our knowledge and experience is this book.

DO CANCER DEFENDERS REALLY WORK?

I'm well aware that Americans have an ingrained skepticism about the idea that the things we eat can make a major difference in the incidence rates of such an awesome disease as cancer. They ask why they haven't heard about these effects all their lives, if a nutritional approach really works. The answer to that shrewd question is that no one knew the facts with any high level of certainty until about 10 years ago. In this relatively short span, the total weight of evidence has reached critical mass. We know now that diet is probably the biggest single influence on cancer. We have thousands of medical studies that support this conclusion. Anyone who examines the evidence carefully and with an open mind will have a difficult time avoiding it.

Here, then, is another simple question, the answer to which holds the entire meaning of this book: What happens to your body if you eat enough broccoli trees and cabbage bunches, carrots and tomatoes, soy foods, fish oils, onions, apples, garlic, mushrooms, ginseng, ginger, vitamins, minerals, cereal grasses, cups of green tea, and a fair sampling of the few dozen other things I'm going to be telling you about? Does your body actually *change?* I know that it does.

Your body politely says, "Thank you," and begins to live at a far higher level of health and energy than most of the other bodies around you.

Moreover, when treated this way, your body builds up a formidable capacity to crush cancers. Crushing cancers is a big part of its proper business. Focus for a moment on one major point: a healthy body *must* crush cancer cells because there are *always* cancer cells at large. Biochemical accidents create malignant and pre-malignant cells daily. To defeat every last one of these dangerous accidents, your body requires world-class defenses. What you're holding in your hands right now is a handbook of cancer defense. Do you need it? Well, just consider the evidence I'm about to give you.

HERE'S THE SITUATION, FOLKS

In 1996, the World Health Organization (WHO) estimated that 10 million new cases of cancer occurred around the world in that year alone. They've predicted that by the year 2001, the number will reach 14.7 million. Meanwhile, in the United States, the rate of cancer mortality was 6 percent higher in 1994 than in 1970. There has been some statistical improvement in the years since, but hardly enough, I'm afraid, to alter the general picture. Approximately every other man and every third woman will get cancer in their lifetime in the United States, if those rates hold up.

Apparently, if there is a war on cancer, our strategies are sorely in need of improvement. Right now, the armies of malignancy have us on the run. This is not surprising, considering the century we live in and our inadequate responses—so far—to the threats that surround us. What we put in our bodies, the way we live our lives and, ultimately, I'm afraid, the way we treat our planet will play a role in our risk for cancer. Because of the nature of cancer, *the best cure for cancer by far is never to get it.*

Almost every cancer patient I've ever treated would have gladly gone back in a time machine to a moment decades before and changed his or her diet and lifestyle if the choice had been offered.

Diet is believed to be the major cause of 30 to 70 percent of all cancers—and this high figure does not include the many cancers attributable to other causes that could have been stopped by proper nutrition.

Consider here these curious facts. Although the incidence of smoking in Japan is almost twice that in America the incidence of lung cancer there is only half as high. The incidence of breast cancer in Japan is one sixth that for American women. The incidence of fatal prostate cancer is one thirtieth that of American men—yes, one thirtieth! In this book, we will show evidence that the consumption of green tea, seaweed, and soy all contribute to the low incidence of cancer in Japan.

The Japanese cancer miracle—for such it might be called—is a small part of the total phytonutrient picture. Hundreds of population studies measuring disease incidence in large populations—we call that the science of epidemiology—show that people who eat the most fruits and vegetables have the greatest ability to detoxify the harmful substances that all of us eat, breathe, or are otherwise exposed to.

As a living creature, you are subject to both internal and external poisoning. You suffer a considerable degree of toxic damage just from the normal, natural workings of your metabolism. You are certainly poisoned by a wide variety of substances, both natural and unnatural, that get into you from outside. Living, even under the best of circumstances, is an enormous physical stress. Your body encounters viruses, toxins, and inflammatory agents on a daily basis. It must deal with these marauders quickly and efficiently.

In many people, I'm afraid, this protective process fails. In the next chapter, I'll discuss the stages by which a cancer is initiated, promoted, and finally threatens your continued existence. Here, I want to make a few general observations about the whole *detoxification* process. What is the basis of success and failure in your private, personal, and unique body?

Let's consider an analogy. You have trillions of cells; in essence you are a metabolic city far larger than any actual city, and like a city, you must produce and consume energy, transport materials and citizens, eliminate trash, handle criminals, and, generally, maintain order and promote the general welfare. Without sufficient power plants, drainage pipes, sanitation trucks, fire engines, police cars, supermarkets, and water mains, the whole vast enterprise would begin to come unhinged. If someone were to introduce poison gas into the mass transit system, as I remember some very strange individuals attempted to do in Tokyo, everything might come permanently to a stop.

Now, we won't need to return to this analogy again, because it really relates to every aspect of human health, and our focus is on cancer. The point is that like a city, your body must have sufficient equipment and hard-working citizens to continue functioning. Cancer is an indication that part of what I should probably call the sanitation system of your multitrillion-cell metropolis has been subpar for quite a while.

Your body needs to clean out dangerous and damaging garbage on a constant basis. It's a vast, thankless enterprise. Without your phytonutrient cleanup brigade, you would soon be neck deep in the big mucky. You wouldn't be detoxified; you would be downright toxic.

In very simple terms, this is why cancer occurs: the body has more toxins than it's capable of processing, cellular damage begins to accumulate, and eventually the situation is serious and perhaps irreversible unless harsh measures are taken.

People will often ask:

- Aren't some people more prone to cancer than others?
- Isn't there such a thing as a genetic predisposition to cancer?
- Isn't cancer fundamentally a disease of aging, as unavoidable as death and taxes?

There is some truth to all those points, and yet cancer is far from unavoidable. Why, for instance, do a significant percentage of genetically very high risk individuals never get cancer? Much of the answer clearly lies in diet and lifestyle.

There's a concept in environmental medicine called "total load." Our bodies are exposed to a wide variety of carcinogenic pollutants daily. Examples are the benzoprene found in cigarette and cigar smoke; the lead and gasoline vapors of industrial and automotive emissions; and the pesticides, herbicides, and hormones that infiltrate our food supply. We also have an internal production of toxic substances caused by metabolizing well-cooked red meat, such preservatives as nitrosamines, and excessive amounts of protein. Added to this total load are various intangible factors, such as the amount of stress and anxiety we're put under. They may increase the toxic load, and they certainly affect the ability of our immune system to handle it.

No one is without a total load of carcinogenic toxicity. In sum, it is the pressure toward cancer that your body labors under. That pressure is always counterbalanced by defenses. If you manage to keep your toxic load in the lower range while building up your phytonutrient defenses to a high level, then whatever your genetic makeup, your chance of getting cancer is small. If the invaders and the defenders are roughly in balance, then the question of whether you'll ever get cancer is a toss-up—you are perhaps an average person. If you have exposed yourself to an enormous toxic load and are doing little to defend yourself, then you are inviting catastrophe—and most often the invitation is accepted.

REAPING THE ENVIRONMENTAL WHIRLWINDS

Let's take a brief detour into the wilderness of our poisoned environment. I simply want to remind you that cancer protection is indeed necessary.

The toxic load we suffer under is neither mythical nor hypothetical.

In the early 1960s, Rachel Carson, by demonstrating the ability of environmental chemicals to disrupt hormones in wildlife, made a revelation, then largely scoffed at, that we were poisoning our planet. She cited many scientific studies showing that the insecticide DDT (dichlorodiphenyltrichloroethane) caused multiple abnormalities in the eggshells of many birds and caused gross deformities in the reproductive organs of many other animals. Some areas replete with a variety of wildlife were decimated by pesticides that filtered through the entire ecosystem. Bald eagles, condors, alligators, and weasels developed disastrous deformities and their populations declined markedly. Carson warned that toxic substances that had such detrimental effects on bird and animal ecosystems might well have similar—if not more profound—effects on humans.

Carson's 1962 best-seller, *Silent Spring*, predicted the global consequences of environmental pollution. The chemical industry spent large sums of money attacking her credibility. Thus, her warning—that what we were doing to our planet we were also doing to ourselves—went largely unheeded. DDT was ultimately banned in the United States in 1973 chiefly because of its obviously devastating impact on wildlife. A concentrated effort to control or even to evaluate the plethora of pesticidal poisons contaminating our food was never made.

Now, consider these eleven facts:

- Hormonelike chemicals found in residues of plastics, pesticides, and petroleum have been found in animals and birds with developmental defects caused by abnormal hormonal function.

- Overexposure to environmental toxins have resulted in two new medical syndromes identified in the 1990s: multiple-chemical sensitivity and sick-building syndrome. Pesticides, heavy metals, and solvents have been implicated in these syndromes by causing damage to the neurologic immune, and endocrine systems.

- Craig Dees and his co-workers at the Oak Ridge National Laboratories in Tennessee have demonstrated that red dye number 3, a common food colorant, markedly increased the proliferation of a human breast cancer cell line that contains estrogen receptors.

- Ana Soto, Ph.D., and her colleagues at Tufts University in Medford, Massachusetts, have demonstrated that certain combinations of environmental chemicals that have contaminated many U.S. rivers can increase breast cancer cell proliferation.

- A study from Michigan demonstrated that women exposed to polychlorinated biphenyl (PCB)-contaminated milk had a twofold excess of breast cancer.

- One hundred fifty billion pounds of prohibited pesticides, such as DDT and chlordane, is shipped out from the United States each year to Third World countries. It comes back to our supermarkets on tropical and "out of season" produce. The U.S. Food and Drug Administration (FDA) Total Diet Survey has found by sampling that DDE (dichlorodiphenyl-dichloroethylene) or DDT contaminates a significant percentage of lamb chops, spinach, raisins and cheddar cheese in this country. Eventually, we will no doubt discover these pesticides in a good many other foods and places, especially since they are capable of evaporating into the atmosphere and condensing when they reach a cooler climate.

- Derva Lee Davis, Ph.D., of the World Resources Institute, Washington, D.C., wrote an article published in the 1994 *Journal of the American Medical Association.* In it, she noted that men and women born in the 1940s had, respectively, twice as much and 30 percent more non–smoking-related cancers as did their ancestors born in the 1890s. She believed environmental toxins play a partial role in this trend.

- Since 1976, the Environmental Protection Agency (EPA) has been measuring toxins from fatty tissue of both autopsies and patients undergoing elective surgery in the United States. Twenty toxic compounds, including OCDD (a dioxin), styrene, 1,4-dichlorobenzene, xylene, toluene, DDE, and PCBs, were found in over 75 percent of all samples.

- Organochlorine metabolites from pesticides and herbicides, such as DDE, oxychlordane, heptachlor epoxide, and dieldrin, were found in 100 percent of fatty tissue samples taken from people in north Texas.

- Mary Wolff, Ph.D., of Mount Sinai School of Medicine in New York has shown that increased serum levels of DDE and PCB is associated with a fourfold increased risk of breast cancer. Organochlorine pesticides, such as hexachlorocyclohexane, DDT, and DDE, have also been found to occur in significantly higher levels in fatty tissue of women with breast cancer than in those without.

- A Swedish study of patients with a blood cancer called multiple myeloma revealed that a prime risk factor, especially among farmers, was exposure to the herbicide chlorophenoxyacid (2,4-D) and the pesticide DDT. Exposure to 2,4-D has also been found to be associated with the development of soft-tissue sarcomas in children, as well as cancers of the stomach and lung and Hodgkin's and non-Hodgkin's lymphomas in adults.

These studies bear out the truth predicted over 100 years ago by Native American Chief Seattle, who wrote: "This, we know: The earth does not belong to us. We belong to the earth. The earth is our mother. What befalls the earth befalls all the sons and daughters of the earth."

YOU'RE IN THE LINE OF FIRE

What I've just offered is only a brief and superficial glance at our cancer–pollution nexus. What it means, of course, is that even those of us who don't smoke, don't eat a high-fat diet, and don't work in a chemical plant are still living, at work and at play, on a profoundly soiled and carcinogenic planet. You may or may not find this alarming, but I think you will readily agree with the advisability of taking steps to defend yourself.

This book is a comprehensive, leading-edge nutritional guide to cancer prevention. If you follow its program, not only will you notice a measurable increase in your sense of health and well-being but you will also definitely lower your probability of ever having to sit across the desk from physicians who refer to themselves as oncologists.

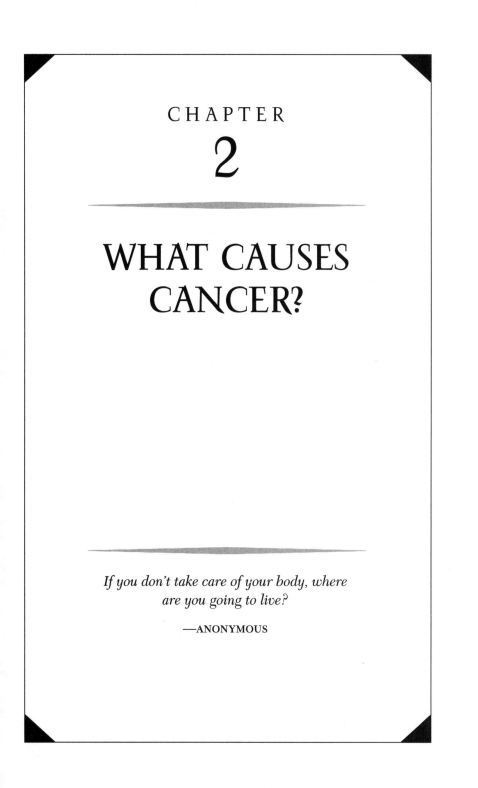

CHAPTER

2

WHAT CAUSES CANCER?

*If you don't take care of your body, where
are you going to live?*

—ANONYMOUS

Cancer? What is this strange development in the human body that strikes fear into the hearts of almost everyone? Have you noticed that some people won't even talk about it? They regard having this terrible and complex disorder as the equivalent of being sentenced to lengthy and unutterable suffering with death for a chaser. This is a disease so stark that folks would rather not speak its name, yet cancer is a largely preventable illness. To regard it in that light rather than elevating it to the status of an unspeakable bogeyman is a much more sensible and health-promoting approach.

So, once again, what exactly is cancer?

Cancer is a family or group of diseases that occur in all human and animal populations (with the interesting exception of sharks) and that may arise in any tissue of the body that is composed of potentially dividing cells. The cells in which cancer occurs show two characteristics. They no longer exhibit normal growth but instead grow uncontrollably, and they no longer carry out the specific body tasks for which cells normally exist but instead simply function as cancer cells. Dividing and multiplying, the cancer cells transmit these characteristics to their cellular offspring. As the cancer grows, the host animal suffers adverse effects caused by invasive growth in the original tumor site or by metastatic spread to other sites in the body.

Cancer is derived from the Greek word *karkinos*, which means "crab." Early physicians noted that the extensive collection of veins surrounding breast tumors look like the claws of a crab. Cancer in humans significantly predates the dawn of civilization. Traces of bone cancer were found in a Javanese skeleton over 1 million years old. Even so, it is probable that in the very worst possible sense, we have come a long way since then. It is now believed that this dis-

17

ease will be the leading cause of death among all age groups by the year 2000. What was once very rare is now very common.

If we don't think about cancer, talk about its causes, and address them, then an appallingly high percentage of all of us—you and me, our loved ones, friends, spouses, children—will be at risk of falling prey to it. We have the evidence to show that extensive lifestyle interventions in the form of nutrition, exercise, and stress reduction can radically cut this cancer surge.

Cancer is now the second leading cause of death in the United States. There were just over 1 million new cases and 500,000 deaths in 1990. Heart disease is the mortality leader, of course, causing 38 percent of all deaths; cancer causes 20 percent. A tragic side note to this is the fact that cancer kills more children than does any other single disease.

Currently, Americans have a one in three chance of developing cancer and a one in six chance of dying of it. The disease reaches into three of every four families, and therefore most people have known a close relative who has battled it. Between 1950 and 1985, there was a 37 percent increase in cancer incidence among Caucasians and an even larger increase among African Americans. The most common cancer in Western countries is lung cancer, followed in descending order by colon and rectal cancer, prostate cancer, and pancreatic cancer.

IN HARM'S WAY

Cancer is such an extraordinarily strange and unexpected process—some part of your own body growing uncontrollably until it harms you—that we need to discuss why it begins and how it progresses.

The first thing to realize is that just simply existing—under the best of physical conditions and with the smallest number of physical stresses—is a far from perfectly benign state of affairs. The effect of being alive, of owning and operating a metabolism that breathes and eats and digests and excretes, is to expose us to dangers and to continuous microscopic harm. Some malignancy-promoting damage is inevitable, therefore, and because it is, our bodies are designed to vigorously defend us.

To understand these basic, inescapable dangers, you need to understand a process called oxidation. You see, oxygen, the very basis of life without which we couldn't live five minutes, much less move, think, and reproduce, also harms us.

In the 1950s, Denham Harman, Ph.D., proposed the antioxidant theory of aging. Dr. Harman had noticed that radiation damaged the human body in ways very similar to the ultimate effects of aging. Excessive radiation exposure was, in fact, an enormously speeded-up equivalent of the daily wear and tear of living and breathing. If this was true, Harman reasoned, then daily living must be a slowed-down version of radiation exposure. He was right, as innumerable studies have since proved.

In carrying out our normal metabolic processes, oxygen oxidizes fuel from the food we eat to produce energy. As a by-product of this oxidation, highly reactive forms of oxygen called free radicals are produced. When molecules in our cells encounter these free radicals, they can suffer serious damage, even to the point of breaking apart.

If you've studied chemistry, you'll recall that a molecule is composed of two or more atoms held together by electron bonds. The electrons are paired, and there is a balanced electrical charge that creates a stable molecular structure. Now, on reacting with oxygen, many molecules gain or lose an electron and become electrically unbalanced. In effect, they become electron hungry. Such molecules are referred to as free radicals. They will vigorously pursue any other molecules they can find and will combine with (that is, oxidize) them. A billionth of a second is all the time a free radical needs to do just that. In making such combinations, free radicals damage the molecules they combine with and, in turn, damage the cells in your body, and that includes damaging their DNA (deoxyribonucleic acid), the material in the nucleus of every cell that contains the genetic program of life. Moreover, every free-radical reaction sets off further free-radical reactions in a geometric chain reaction. In effect, free radicals wildly reproduce themselves.

Trillions of these reactions (to say the least) are occurring in our bodies daily. In fact, it has been estimated that every cell in our bodies takes 10,000 oxidative hits to its DNA daily. We would soon succumb to this barrage if not for the defense given us by our own team of antioxidants, some produced in our body but the vast majority provided by the nutrients, especially by the phytonutrients, in our daily diet. As Bruce Ames, Ph.D., one of the leading experts on cancer in America, has remarked, not to eat fruits and vegetables is the equivalent of irradiating yourself!

Antioxidant metabolism explains a great deal of the process of cancer. Most of the risk factors for cancer are in one way or another related to an increased rate of free-radical attack on the cells of the body. This includes smoking, excessive unprotected exposure to sunlight, exposure to poisonous chemicals in our food and environment, and even many forms of infection and inflammation that promote cancer. Since most of the phytonutrients that I will discuss in this book are potent antioxidants, it is clear that we find ourselves involved in a very real metabolic war—with the free-radical attackers paired off against our antioxidant defenders. Now with this information under our belts, let's look at the stages a person travels through if he or she is attacked by cancer.

NOT ALL AT ONCE BUT STEP BY STEP

The cancer process can be simplified into the following sequence of steps:

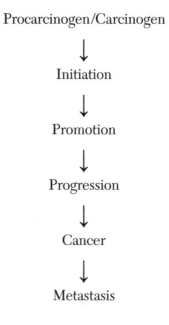

Procarcinogen/Carcinogen

↓

Initiation

↓

Promotion

↓

Progression

↓

Cancer

↓

Metastasis

There are three basic levels here:

- The level of initiation of cell damage by carcinogens or pro-carcinogens
- The level of promotion and progression toward a clinically definable cancer state
- The level of indisputable cancer and its spread (metastasis) to other areas of the body

Different factors cause, promote, or maintain the cancer process at each of these levels. Some factors, such as smoking, may play a role at more than one stage.

Any chemical agent that initiates the cancer process is a carcinogen or procarcinogen. All around us in the environment are such initiators as PCBs (polychlorinated biphenyls), diverse pesticides, dioxin, petroleum-based products, cooking and heating fumes, cigarette smoke (both first- and secondhand) and ultraviolet (UV) radiation from the sun. These high-risk initiators might be considered to be over and above the cancer-inducing effects of normal metabolism, the pro-oxidant processes that we outlined above in our discussion of free-radical pathology.

Procarcinogens are distinct from carcinogens simply because in order to exert a carcinogenic effect, they need the assistance of activating enzymes found right in our own bodies. Without that assistance, they remain harmless. Benzoprene, for instance, a major chemical by-product of smoking, is not a carcinogen in its own right, but if it becomes activated by enzymes in the body to produce benzoprene epoxide, the resulting compound is very potently carcinogenic. Therefore, nutrients that block the activity of benzoprene-converting enzymes (green tea is an outstanding example, as is curcumin, the active ingredient in curry powder) also may partially inhibit some of the DNA-damaging effects of smoking.

Once initiation has occurred—which implies that permanent damage to the DNA of some cells has been successfully carried out—there are many factors that can promote continued progress toward carcinoma. Our own sex hormones appear to have this effect in certain areas of the body. Chronic inflammation or infection may promote cancer. High-fat diets based on the wrong kinds of fats (see Chapter 7) are suspected to be promoters of a variety of cancers, especially breast cancers, colorectal cancers, and prostate cancers. Alcohol (for breast and liver cancer) and polyunsaturated fats can also be effective promoters. High-carbohydrate diets rich in sugar and other refined starches seem to be associated with breast cancer because of their effect on insulin levels, and their interaction with estrogen receptor sites.

Having gotten this far, let's look at cancer at the level where it all begins, the individual cell.

JUST WHAT HAPPENS IN A CANCEROUS CELL?

You have over 100 trillion cells in your body. Considering the assault they're under, the remarkable thing about the human body is the complete efficiency with which it will usually suppress cancer. Your body is custom designed to prevent malignancies. It is a cancer-crushing machine.

Yet cancers do start—at the cellular level. Cancer cells are very different from the normal cells in your body. Let me tell you what happens as a cell matures. Fresh, young cells in their immature state have not yet been fitted out to perform necessary activities in the body; they are what physicians call undifferentiated. As these cells differentiate, they have "career paths" chosen for them from which, henceforth, they will never deviate. It is similar to a person's being trained at a certain age to be a carpenter or an automobile mechanic, a doctor or a lawyer, a cook or a soldier, with no possibility thereafter of that person becoming anything different—once the mold is set, the profession is in place until death. This is the way it is with your cells. They differentiate into their separate "career paths" as nerve cells or muscle cells, bone cells, digestive cells, or whatever the case may be.

To begin with, though, new cells are more malleable. It is these youthful, undifferentiated cells that most typically become cancerous. As a result, they never do mature—they never take up a "profession," they never serve a useful function, they never differentiate. Their job, in fact, is to grow and multiply as part of a rebel cancer colony. In that role, they will bring disorder to your body and, just possibly, terminal chaos. Because of their lack of differentiation, they are readily identifiable under the microscope and are called anaplastic. This comes from the Greek words *ana,* meaning "prior to" and *plasia,* meaning "form." Many of these cells also have certain proteins on their surfaces that differentiated cells do not; these tend to be released into the bloodstream, and there are lab tests to detect them.

There are other patterns of abnormal cellular growth that warn of the possibility of cancer. *Dysplasia,* which means "abnormal form," refers to cells that mature in a disorganized way. The condition indicates a strong probability of future cancer in the area examined. Dysplasia can be readily identified by medical specialists. Dysplasia of cells in the cervical lining is picked up by a routine Pap (Papanicolaou) smear—a procedure developed at the Strang Center—and is a clear warning that cervical cancer may eventually occur. Another prime location for investigation for dysplasia is the cells lining the bronchial tubes of the lung. These cells can be coughed up in the sputum and examined. Should they be dysplastic, this would be referred to as bronchial dysplasia. It is a risk factor for the imminent development of lung cancer.

Two other disorders of cell plasia, or form, are worth briefly examining. *Hyperplasia* refers to an increased number of cells, usually in diseases of the breast or uterine lining. If anaplasia or dysplasia are also found, this finding is especially worrisome.

Let's Have a Little Differentiation Around Here!

It is also important to note that the lack of differentiation characteristic of cells that are moving down the assembly line toward carcinogenesis is not irreversible. Many types of cancer cells can be induced to differentiate to a less malignant form by exposure to various nutrients. Some of the phytonutrients found in vegetables have been shown to induce the differentiation of cells of the head, neck, and lung, as well as to promote differentiation of leukemia cells.

Most important of all, it has been demonstrated repeatedly in both animal and human studies that dietary changes can actually reverse premalignant changes in many different sites in the body. Cells that have begun to turn cancerous can return to functionality.

Some nutrients display the ability to influence cellular differentiation. References are made in this text to many of these nutrients.

Metaplasia refers to a situation in which one type of normal lining tissue changes into another. For instance, in Barrett's esophagus, a condition that causes repeated episodes of heartburn, there is a cellular change of the tissue in the esophagus that can be discovered by testing. Such a change is associated with a high risk for esophageal carcinoma. (Please note that not all habitual heartburn indicates cancer, but all such symptoms should be checked.)

All these different plasias represent aspects of progression toward a clinically definable cancer state. Once that state occurs, meaning that cancer cells with damaged DNA and abnormal form are present, they will be attacked by various cells in our immune systems, such as natural killer cells, mononuclear cells, and polymorphonuclear cells. The fighting ability of all these cells of the immune system is enhanced by a variety of important phytonutrients, which we will be explaining nutrient by nutrient throughout the book.

As we're about to see, however, phytonutrients can also prevent cells from ever reaching a cancerous stage.

Blocking and Suppressing Those Cancer Cells

To a certain extent, most carcinogens are actually procarcinogens and require metabolic activation of some kind if they are to progress on toward cancer. Blocking agents in our food can prevent them from becoming active in a cancerous way.

Several kinds of vegetables are particularly rich in these blocking agents. Such cruciferous vegetables as cabbage, broccoli, brussels sprouts, turnips, and mustard greens are outstanding examples. Garlic is rich in sulfur-containing blocking agents, as are its relatives, onions, leeks, and shallots. Citrus fruit oils contain yet another variety of blocking agent, two of which—D-limonene and D-carvone—have been investigated and found effective. D-carvone is also found in caraway seed oil.

All of the above agents increase the activity of detoxifying enzymes that are employed by the body to break down active carcinogens before they can damage the DNA of cells. These are the Phase 2 enzymes that will be discussed in much greater detail in Chapter 4.

In addition to the blocking agents, your phytonutrient protection brigade contains suppressing agents that stop the development of already damaged cells and suppress the growth of what would have turned out to be cancerous tissue. Much less is known about suppressing agents, and not too many of them have been identified. We do know, however, that some suppressors are found in cruciferous vegetables.

Chapter by chapter, then, in the rest of the book, I will demonstrate just how effective plant food is in blocking carcinogens.

The above is, of course, an elementary description of a complicated and variable process. Let's look now at some of the carcinogens and precarcinogens that lead to the initiation of a cancer. For clarity's sake, they are divided into four main groups.

CHEMICALS

In 1800, it was observed that miners who had prolonged contact with coal and tar had a high incidence of lung cancer. Early in the twentieth century, benzoprene was identified as a major carcinogen; it is found in coal and tar, as well as in cigarette smoke. When it and other related aromatic hydrocarbons were applied directly to the skin of laboratory animals, cancers formed.

Chemical carcinogens are exceedingly prevalent in our environment, even if you avoid tobacco smoke. The food additives nitrites turn into carcinogenic nitrosamines in your body; petroleum-based products are high-risk entities; some of the pesticides that our food is sprayed with have cancer promoting effects—but many others have not been adequately tested. There are natural carcinogenic chemicals as well, such as the aflatoxin found in corn and peanuts—and that includes peanut butter; you might want to try almond butter or cashew butter for a healthier snack. Scientists have estimated that, in general, environmental factors—including smoking and diet—are responsible for 70 to 80 percent of all cancers.

IONIZING RADIATION

It is well known that UV radiation from the sun is one of the major contributing risk factors of skin cancer. It is also well known that exposure to X-rays and gamma rays contribute to leukemia, lymphoma, and thyroid and bone cancer. Radiation exposure has caused a higher incidence of leukemia and breast cancer in Japanese survivors of the atom bomb blast. Statistics also show that people who work around medical X-rays or in nuclear power plants have somewhat higher risk of contracting these cancers.

Therefore, you need to be aware of the possible sources of radiation in your life. For instance, it is up to you to ask if the X-rays you are receiving really serve a useful purpose. Do you need a chest X-ray every year? It's for you and your doctor to decide. As a consumer, you should always ask your dentist if "routine" dental X-rays are absolutely necessary. Is he or she using the modern dental X-ray machines that minimize X-ray exposure? If your dentist isn't, see if you can convince him or her that obtaining such equipment is necessary for maintaining patient loyalty, including yours. Lowering your lifetime exposure to radiation must be your basic goal. Your cumulative exposure over years and decades is what may get you into trouble and what you are trying to minimize.

Recently, across the country, the press has paid much attention to the gas radon and the threat it poses to the health of home owners. This gas, produced by the natural breakdown of radium or uranium, is a fairly serious radiation risk factor for the development of lung cancer. Radon may be present in rocks and soil beneath a house. Released as a vapor, it seeps through cracks in basement floors or travels up pipes that come up from deep wells. The happy home owner sitting in an armchair reading a newspaper has little idea that he or she is being steadily irradiated.

The highest levels of radon are found in New Jersey, Pennsylvania, Colorado, Florida, and New Hampshire. The Environmental Protection Agency (EPA) has found that approximately 12 percent of American homes contained elevated levels of radon; that is, levels higher than four picocuries of radon per liter of air. Radon detection kits can be purchased at most hardware stores. If you find elevated levels, you can contact the local office of the EPA and ask for a list of certified radon abatement specialists who can evaluate your home. Radon abatement usually involves sealing up all the cracks in your basement, which usually lowers levels by approximately 80 percent, or running a pipe under the foundations, sucking the vapors up, and blowing them out above the house, where they dissipate quite nicely.

Another radiation risk factor that we can certainly all take steps against is UV light. This is a serious matter because we are now being exposed to more of it. Depletion of the ozone layer by the chlorofluorocarbons (CFCs)—substances present in aerosol sprays, air conditioners, and most refrigerant systems—is causing more UV radiation to penetrate our atmosphere.

Here are four steps that you can take to minimize your lifelong exposure to UV radiation:

- Avoid getting a sunburn at any time in your life. If you have children, take steps to protect them. It is well documented that even one major sunburn—especially one in which blisters occurs—markedly increases your lifetime risk of developing the deadliest form of skin cancer: melanoma.
- Remember that UV rays are present even when there is no direct sun exposure. Just because it's cloudy out is no reason not to protect yourself. In addition, people who enjoy winter sports ought to wear sunscreen and appropriate skin coverings because snow (and, in summertime, sand) reflects UV rays. Cover your skin surfaces as thoroughly as possible. Include brimmed hats and shirts with a collar and long sleeves in your wardrobe.
- Sunscreens are important and should have an SPF (solar protection factor) of more than 15. It is important to apply sunscreen at least every 2 to 3 hours if you are being directly exposed to the sun.
- Avoid prolonged exposure to UV light even if you are taking all of the above precautions. Remember that the most intense exposure is between 10 A.M. and 2 P.M.; find a shady spot. The many people who have started going to artificial tanning salons should also be concerned. Quite simply, we do not know what long-range risks are associated with this type of exposure. UV light is made up of ultraviolet A (UVA) and ultraviolet B (UVB) rays. It is believed that the UVB rays are more carcinogenic. The tanning machines tend to use more UVA light, but on the downside, this light penetrates deeper

into the skin and the tan produced does not seem to provide as much protection against UV sun damage as a tan achieved with sunlight. In addition, the relatively noncarcinogenic character of UVA has been called into question by studies in animals that show it causes skin cancer and premature aging. The bottom line? Avoid tanning salons.

INFECTIONS

Cancer researchers now estimate that infection may account for up to 10 percent of all cancers. For instance, a virus called human T-cell lymphoma virus 1 (HTLV-1) causes T-cell lymphoma. Another virus called HTLV-2 causes a type of leukemia called hairy-cell leukemia. In some people, the Epstein-Barr virus appears to promote Burkitt's lymphoma, a cancer mostly associated with the continent of Africa. This virus has also been found in some lymphomas occurring in patients with acquired immunodeficiency syndrome (AIDS) as well as in cancers of the nose found in Cantonese Chinese. Herpesvirus and human papillomaviruses (HPVs) have been implicated in the development of cervical cancer. Liver cancer is also strongly associated with the hepatitis virus. For this reason, it's probable that the worldwide use of hepatitis B vaccine can prevent more than 90 percent of all cases of liver cancer. Finally, a bacteria, *Helicobacter pylori,* has been found to be a causative agent of both stomach cancer and lymphomas of the stomach. The treatment of *Helicobacter pylori* (a simple antibiotic regimen) can cause some types of stomach lymphoma to disappear without the need for chemotherapy, radiation, or surgery.

DIET

High-fat diets are strongly associated with two common cancers—colorectal and prostate—and somewhat more hypothetically related to breast cancer. The exact mechanism by which fat promotes cancer still needs to be worked out, but the epidemiologic evidence is quite strong. Much of that evidence, however, could indicate the risks of diets low in plant food just as readily as it could represent the risks of fat. We're not really sure which risk is more significant. Particularly in the case of colorectal cancer, an inadequate intake of fiber may be the most crucial component. Further tips on good fats and bad fats will be found in Chapter 7. For an extensive discussion of fiber, see Chapter 18.

Another dietary risk is the toxic overload of hormones and pesticides found in our food. Shopping organic is a very smart move. My family and I buy organic milk, produce, and natural meat; natural meat, for example, is currently being marketed without hormones or antibiotics, and beef from Argentina is now being shipped into this country that is taken from free-range cattle fed in wide open pastures and not pumped up with growth hormone or other antibiotics. Bug your local supermarket manager. The market will soon start selling these meat cuts.

DON'T PUT YOURSELF AT RISK

Most of the above factors are to some extent controllable. It is certainly possible to refrain from smoking, although it is difficult to stop once you begin. It is reasonable and not too financially burdensome to eat organic food. Exposure to UV light can be minimized. Infections can be treated, diet can be changed, common sense can be maximized.

Better than 90 percent of all cancers are represented in the categories above. All of these cancers—as well as the other 10 percent—almost universally respond (often by never occurring in the first place) to a fruit- and vegetable-driven diet, a cuisine soaked in phytonutrients, a green revolution occurring inside you.

By taking reasonable precautions against cancer, cardiovascular disease, and accidents, we can prolong our lives beyond anything thought possible only a few decades ago, and those will be lives well worth living, for their extended length in years will showcase the remarkable fact of their enhanced quality.

CHAPTER 3

YOUR INCOMPARABLE IMMUNE SYSTEM

*What you should put first in all the
practice of our art is how to make the
patient well; and if he [or she] can be made
well in many ways, one should choose the
least troublesome.*

—HIPPOCRATES

I n this chapter and the one that follows, I am going to briefly explain two of the body's major cancer protection systems. Your immune system and your liver are hard at work, from the time you're born till the time you die, eliminating a host of deadly threats to your existence. Once you've seen how well they work, it will be easy to appreciate the absolute importance of supporting them with a massive daily dose of phytonutrients. In many ways, you're about to look into the nitty-gritty of cancer defense.

Within you are all the elements of a fully functioning department of defense. Like citizen-soldiers, the cells of your immune system quickly march in their millions and tens of millions to any site of infection and slaughter the invaders. They have guards posted to spot the first sign of trouble, they have a communications network, they have commanders who decide who they'll attack and who is in possession of the password and therefore free to come or go. They have army bases where the troops stay when they're not fighting, they have the ability to explosively multiply their numbers—the equivalent of a draft instituted during the direst emergency—and they declare peace and partly demobilize after the war is won. They have determination, self-sacrifice, and the will to win.

Malignant cells are one of the things this highly aggressive standing army has the ability and the desire to destroy. I'd like us to take a closer look at the immune system before we wander through the incredible variety of cancer-preventive foods, herbs, and supplements.

THE NATURAL IMMUNE SYSTEM

To continue with the military metaphor, your immune system is equipped to face threats from land, sea, and air. Let the assault come against skin, mucous membranes, blood, lungs, digestive tract, or any other imaginable interior or exterior body surface; your immune system will be there. Its duties include not only trapping and killing infections but recognizing and destroying damaged or mutated cells.

We generally divide the immune system's activities into two parts. We speak of the "natural" immune system and the "acquired" immune system. The natural immune system is our first line of defense, the various cells that attack any and all intruders on every occasion they appear. The acquired immune system is a somewhat more sophisticated operation that learns to target very specific invaders.

The natural immune system is quite a grab bag of defenders. Our skin itself, our tears, our ear wax, our mucus all have ways of inhibiting and destroying infectious organisms like viruses and bacteria. Inside us, a formidable array of cellular defenders stand ready to attack. First, there are the phagocytes, large white blood cells that engulf and literally digest invading bacteria, as well as any of our own cells that seem to have suffered damage. Then there are natural killer cells.

Natural killer cells are one of the body's first defenses against cancer. These very large immune system assassins are often called granulocytes because they're filled with granules that contain a variety of chemical weapons suitable for the destruction of malignant cells. I'm sure you recall how I said earlier that the average cell suffers 10,000 free-radical assaults per day. Good antioxidant protection saves most of those cells from serious damage. The cells that don't make it through the barrage, however—the ones that come out changed, mutated, Dr. Jekylls turned into Mr. Hydes— these the immune system hunts down and the natural killer cell execution teams finish off. As I've said elsewhere, our body is powerfully programmed to crush cancers.

The natural immune system, then, shows a gargantuan and relatively undiscriminating appetite for anything that appears to be alien.

THE ACQUIRED IMMUNE SYSTEM

The acquired immune system is a far more sophisticated team of defenders. It doesn't just send out untrained hordes of cellular fighters to swallow anything that turns up. Instead, it educates professional soldiers, the West Point cadets of the immune system, who learn what to look for.

The acquired immune system has specialist cells called lymphocytes or T-cells, each of which recognizes the molecular code for particular microorganisms. These T-cells originate in our bone marrow, but then they go to our thymus gland to refine and polish their education. Different cells specialize in the recognition of different invaders. One will respond to herpesvirus, another will recognize and violently assault the tuberculosis microbe, a third will lie in wait for the rhinovirus—the common cold.

Once these cells recognize their enemy, they call for more troops. Chemical messages are sent by substances called cytokines informing the body which T-cells are needed for this particular emergency. Within a relatively short period of time, millions of copies of these T-cell killer specialists are manufactured by your immune system and sent to the battlefield armed to the teeth with enough chemical weaponry to turn any general green with envy.

When new infections come our way, microbial invaders that our immune system has never seen before, some clever young officers in the T-cell army learn their molecular code, participate in their destruction, and afterwards *remember* what they've learned. From that point on, the body has specialists that will immediately recognize and assault this invader if it should appear again. The substance—bacteria or virus or whatever it may be—that the body reacts against is called an antigen. The cells that specialize in attacking any specific antigen are called antibodies.

You're still alive, right? This tells you that your unwearying defense forces have won millions of minor skirmishes and hundreds of major battles on your behalf!

BUT NOTHING'S PERFECT

This fiendishly complex and stunningly efficient defense industry of yours can also cause you some trouble. The very systems that act so vigorously to oppose infection or the intrusion of anything at all that your immune system defines as "not you" can overreact. Then they may produce a state of chronic inflammation or, through a breakdown in the system, an attack upon some part of your body.

There are many examples. Such serious conditions as rheumatoid arthritis, lupus, Crohn's disease, and multiple sclerosis are referred to as autoimmune diseases, meaning that the body attacks itself. In other words, the immune system misidentifies normal parts of the body as alien invaders and sets out to destroy them. The complications can be severe.

At other times, the body may overreact to something like pollen, and you have yourself an allergy. It may learn to regard a particular food as an inappropriate and dangerous invader on your intestinal shores, and every time you eat that food, you may experience discomfort or loss of energy without necessarily knowing the cause.

Unfortunately, the activities of a normally vigilant immune system can sometimes lead to cancer. The pathway this follows is usually chronic inflammation. For example, there is the damage caused to the stomach by *Helicobacter pylori*. This bacteria attaches itself to the wall of the stomach or the upper part of the small intestine; by degrading urea into ammonia, it causes intense irritation. In fact, *Helicobacter* is now recognized as one of the major causes of stomach ulcers. It's also suspected that, at least in America, it may be the major culprit in stomach cancer.

In the *Helicobacter*/cancer scenario, what happens is this: The immune system's response to all the irritation and infection occurring in the stomach is vigorous enough to cause severe local inflammation. Over a long period, inflammation can cause equally severe free-radical reactions in cells, leading to mutation and cancer. I'd like you to bear with me now for a few paragraphs as I get a little bit technical. What I'm about to explain is quite important, and it's worth the effort of understanding.

The process of inflammation that we just spoke of is frequently engineered by an enzyme that's very important in cancer studies. This is the cyclooxygenase-2 or COX-2 enzyme, and I'll be referring back to it many times in the course of this book, so let me explain it now. COX-2 stimulates the production of an inflammatory prostaglandin (PGE-2) that the body uses—naturally—to promote inflammation.

The human body works according to a system of balances and counterbalances. Certain chemicals in the body are designed to rev you up and others are designed to put you to sleep; some chemicals will raise your blood pressure and others will lower it. The way that the body achieves an ideal balance—to the extent that it does achieve it—occurs by its manipulation of the chemical signals that raise and lower metabolic functions. Therefore, when we say that too much of something—let's say cholesterol—is bad for you, we don't mean that cholesterol itself is bad for you. In fact, you couldn't live without it: it's one of the major building blocks of the human body.

The same thing is true of prostaglandins, a talented team of hormonelike substances that affect immune response and blood pressure, inhibit certain allergies, and depending on the prostaglandin, provoke or prevent inflammation. There are three main prostaglandins that we'll discuss in this book, numbered 1 to 3. By and large, I'll be advising you to do things that promote the production of PGE-1 and PGE-3 and that lower the levels of PGE-2, the pro-inflammation prostaglandin. That doesn't mean the body made a mistake in designing that particular prostaglandin. Sometimes inflammation is necessary.

For its part, PGE-1 is important in protecting your stomach from too much acid and keeping your kidneys working normally, among other things. This is why people who take too much aspirin can occasionally develop problems with ulcers and kidney disease.

Now, the best method of lowering PGE-2 is usually to keep down your levels of the COX-2 enzyme, its primary stimulator. COX-2 is triggered by a number of situations. Eating too little dietary fat will tend to promote COX-2 activity, and so will eating too much of such common polyunsaturated omega-6 fatty-acids—rich oils as sunflower, safflower, corn, and canola (oils). Yet another way to increase COX-2 is to consume an insufficient amount of the omega-3 fatty acids found in fish, plankton, flaxseed, and hempseed. Chapter 7 is entirely devoted to the oils, so if you want more information on this extremely important aspect of your diet, go there.

In that chapter, I will tell you just what you need to do to keep your PGE-2 down in the lower range. Here are three more reasons why you should:

- The type of inflammation stimulated by PGE-2 is involved in the formation of breast, colon, and prostate cancers.

- PGE-2 is involved in autoimmune disease and plaque buildup in the arteries.
- PGE-2 can inhibit natural killer cell activity, thus disarming the very cells that should hunt out and destroy malignancies.

Your Diet Will Make Your Immune System Hum

In addition to choosing your prostaglandins, you will want to do the utmost to stimulate the overall health of your immune system. A phytonutrient-rich diet, a reasonable amount of exercise, and the avoidance whenever possible of excessive stress is the best combination that I know. Also remember that many very familiar vitamins and minerals aid the immune system in its quest to hunt and kill cancer cells. Here is a sampling of these important aids:

- Vitamins matter. Low intake of vitamin A, beta carotene, B_6, vitamin C, vitamin E, and folic acid has been associated with abnormally low immune response and a greater risk of developing cancer.
- A study of the food records of 62 adults with cancer with early stages of active disease found substantial dietary deficiencies. When their vitamin and mineral intake was compared to population averages (which are themselves inadequate by the standards of this book), they were found to have lower intake of vitamins A, C, D, E, B_1, B_2, B_3, B_6, and B_{12} and the mineral zinc.
- Low levels of zinc allow the thymus gland, one of the immune system's primary sites, to shrink. That's where your body's T-cells go to get their higher education. Zinc supplementation in animals has been shown to stimulate the regrowth of the thymus gland and cause a recovery in the number of T-cells. Elderly people are often low in zinc. This can result from their eating less red meat, from their eating less overall, and from the myriad drug interactions that they may be experiencing. In their case in particular, zinc supplementation may be desirable.
- Selenium, one of your body's micronutrients, has an outstanding and well-deserved reputation as a cancer fighter.

One study of healthy college students found that even with the youthful and presumably vigorous immune systems of this group, selenium could make a difference. The students who were given 200 micrograms of selenium daily had a 118 percent increase in their white blood cells' capacity for killing cancer cells. Moreover, their natural killer cell activity was increased by 82.3 percent.

DON'T BE CAUGHT WITH YOUR IMMUNE SYSTEM DOWN

You can probably see what the rest of this book will amply illustrate. Got an immune system? Go with it. Play to its strengths; minimize its weaknesses. It's your friend. It's your own private army. Its patriotism is unquestionable. It will die for you, and it will kill for you. If you care for it and fund it with phytonutrients, it will be your most valuable ally against most disease dangers, including cancer.

BIG DEFENDERS: YOUR LIVER AND ITS ENZYMES

*The physician's job is to program
people to live.*

—NORMAN COUSINS

Without your liver, you would be toxic soup. By some calculations, this remarkable organ does over 400 different jobs. Unlike those other workhorses—the heart, the lungs, and the digestive tract, which basically do the same job over and over—the liver is an impresario of diversity, a circus showman who always has at least ten acts going at the same time.

This diversity of functions is probably why the liver, weighing in at four pounds, is the largest organ in the body. It has to store vital nutrients; it must produce bile needed for the absorption of fat; it must regulate your blood sugar levels by creating glycogen, a stored form of blood sugar; it must create such fats as cholesterol and most of the soluble proteins in your blood, including albumin; and it assists in the metabolism of thyroid hormones.

Most important of all, it has to dispose of bodily wastes and decide how to process the hundreds of thousands of unnatural bodily chemicals (xenobiotics) that we're increasingly exposed to. This is one workaholic organ that never heard the word *vacation* and has the tenacity of a pit bull.

Sending Those Carcinogens into Exile

We are and must and will be exposed to cancer-causing toxic substances throughout our lives. Therefore, it's obvious that having safe, certain, and speedy methods of getting them out of our bodies after they've gotten in is essential.

Your liver has a number of methods of dealing with toxins. First of all, it has its own SWAT team, squads of macrophages called Kupffer's cells that live in the liver and engulf and annihilate a fair percentage of both the bacterial and toxic substances that come its

43

way. They're a busy bunch, because almost two quarts of blood pass through the liver every minute for detoxification.

Second, the liver manufactures one quart of bile acid a day, and this carries many toxic substances down to the intestines for excretion in your stools. I'll be talking a little more about this system in a moment.

Third, the liver has a two-step enzymatic system for neutralizing xenobiotics and many other substances that need elimination. Just in an average day, your liver might want to bring down the curtain on an assortment of toxins such as the following: old, used-up body hormones, including estrogens and insulin; damaged cholesterol; insecticide residues; prescription drugs; alcohol; ammonia, a by-product of muscular exertion; and various poisons that make their way into your body through the air you breathe, the food you eat, or the water you drink. Your liver is a hard taskmaster, and it will not tolerate the buildup of such toxic refuse.

The enzymatic steps that now occur are called Phase 1 and Phase 2 detoxification. It's a complex and crucial system. Carried out properly, it will swiftly eliminate most chemical carcinogens without too much damage being done to your body. If it's carried out clumsily, inadequately, or with poor synchronization of the two phases, you're in for trouble. Let's look at these two phases closely, and then consider some of the vitamins, minerals, and phytonutrients that promote efficiency.

PHASE 1

Phase 1 uses a detoxification family of enzymes known as the cytochrome P450 system. These break apart many of the chemical bonds holding the toxins together. The process is called hydroxylation. Some of the toxins become more water soluble and many of them, in this phase at least, are made temporarily more chemically active. In a phrase, they are being prepared for Phase 2.

The efficiency of the Phase 1 system varies from individual to individual. There are 50 to 100 enzymes working in the P450 system, and particular enzymes specialize in handling specific toxins. People vary in the degree to which their P450 system is capable of handling this or that poison. It's believed that that's the reason why some people handle the carcinogens in cigarettes very well, chain-smoke for 50 years, and die in their beds of something entirely unrelated to lung cancer. They have reaped the benefits of genetic variability.

PHASE 2

Even as Phase 1 is busy breaking down the toxins that it wants to eliminate while making others more active, phase 2 enzymes are getting ready to carry the process further by attaching various detoxification enzymes to these chemically altered toxins. This process is called conjugation.

Conjugation should occur more or less in sync with Phase 1 hydroxylation. If it lags behind, you can be harmed by the toxins that Phase 1 has released. They're still partly fat soluble, and if they end up getting stored in your fat tissue indefinitely, this could lead to some dire effects. The completion of the Phase 1 process is therefore a moment of some danger. Many toxins are now more carcinogenic and chemically active than they were before detoxification began.

If Phase 1 activation runs ahead of Phase 2 conjugation, then your detoxification pathways overload. The toxins present in that overload can begin to bind with the DNA (deoxyribonucleic acid) in your cells. The results will be cell injury, mutation, and death. For this reason, it's critically important to have enough of the Phase 2 enzymes on hand at all times.

The most important nutrients that support Phase 2 enzymes are sulfate, glucuronic acid, and glutathione (also known as GSH). Of these detoxifying enzymes, glutathione-S-transferase is critically important in almost every organ of the body. People vary in their levels of this enzyme, and research suggests that those with partial deficiencies have a higher risk of lung cancer.

Of the enzyme-supporting nutrients, glutathione is outstanding. It is certainly the most abundant antioxidant in the human body and perhaps the most important. This may surprise you if you've been reading for years about antioxidants and the only names that stuck were vitamin C, vitamin E, and beta carotene. I suppose we don't talk about glutathione that much because most of it is manufactured in the body from protein, something of which there is seldom a shortage in our society, so most vitamin enthusiasts are not concerned about taking glutathione supplements.

There should always be a good deal of glutathione present in the neighborhood of the liver not only because this substance is necessary for Phase 2 conjugation of toxins by such enzymes as quinone reductase, UDP-glucuronyl-transferase, and glutathione-S-transferase but also because your poor, overworked liver is a hot-bed of free-radical activity. Imagine dealing with all those toxic chemicals daily! Naturally, the liver needs some top-quality antioxidants around to mop up free radicals and minimize damage to itself. Glutathione and other enzyme system antioxidants are usually there—or should be.

As a matter of fact, having ample supplies of glutathione is a very serious responsibility for your body and if you look at the next Pharmacist's Corner (page 47), you'll find some suggestions about ensuring a glutathione sufficiency. First, however, if you want to know how important glutathione is, glance at the partial list below.

- Glutathione is a major antioxidant in tissues throughout the body.
- Glutathione rehabilitates such antioxidants as vitamins C and E. Once these vitamins have been busy in your cells scavenging free radicals, they can become oxidized themselves. Glutathione easily restores them to what is called their reduced form so they can get back to work again.
- Glutathione helps in the production, defense, and repair of DNA.
- Glutathione is very stable and has the ability to neutralize free radicals many times before it itself is oxidized. Moreover, it itself can usually be quickly and easily recycled back to a reduced state by other antioxidants in the body.
- Glutathione protects against ultraviolet (UV) damage in certain wavelengths.
- Glutathione improves immune function and, indeed, is abundant in white blood cells.
- Glutathione has a particular capacity for binding and supervising the removal of toxic heavy metals, such as lead, mercury, and arsenic, all of which our modern environment exposes us to.

Pharmacist's Corner

■ **N-acetyl-cysteine (NAC):** take 600 milligrams once daily with food. Studies demonstrate that at this dosage NAC is both safe and effective as an antioxidant and chemopreventive nutrient. Other studies show that at a dosage of 600 milligrams twice daily, NAC helps protect white blood cells, promote proper immune function, and protects you from developing a flu infection. NAC is a major precuressor for the production of glutathione.

■ **Glutathione:** glutathione is available from a number of companies. Although it is difficult to absorb, there is some evidence that in patients with very low glutathione levels, the body has increased ability to absorb this very important detoxifying antioxidant. A good dose of glutathione would be 250 to 500 milligrams daily with food. It is important to note that the mineral selenium and vitamin B_2 are needed for glutathione's antioxidant activity, so it is a good idea to take a glutathione supplement that includes both of these important nutrients if you are not already supplementing with them.

■ **Whey protein:** whey protein contains small amounts of glutathione and L-cysteine. Normally, I do not like L-cysteine because it is unstable and therefore easily oxidized; however, in whey, there are cofactors, such as lactoferrin and lactalbumin, which increase the conversion rate of L-cysteine to glutathione, according to studies from McGill University in Montreal, Quebec, Canada.

■ **Broccoli:** see Chapter 9 (Cruciferous Vegetables).

■ **Citrus oil extract:** take 250 to 500 milligrams once or twice daily with meals. This supplement should contain 85% D-limonene. Note: some people experience indigestion with this supplement.

■ **Green tea:** see Chapter 19 (Green Tea).

■ **Turmeric:** see Chapter 10 (Herbs and Bees).

■ **Indole-3 carbinol:** take from 200 to 600 milligrams daily with a meal.

■ **L-Glutamine;** see Chapter 14, Indole-3 carbinol is an active constituent found in cruciferous vegetables.

■ **Milk thistle:** see Chapter 10 (Herbs and Bees).

■ **Selenium:** See Chapter 16 (Minerals).

SUPPORT PHASE 2 DETOXIFICATION TO HELP PREVENT CANCER

It may seem as if we've gotten a little bit off the subject of this book, which is preventing cancer, but we really are on target. The liver is a major built-in cancer fighter, as important, in its own way, as the immune system. Obviously, therefore, whatever supports its efficient functioning lessens your lifetime risks.

A 1998 study by Kathy Helzlsouer, M.D., M.P.H., and colleagues at Johns Hopkins University School of Public Health in Baltimore, published in the *Journal of the National Cancer Institute,* compared the genetic detoxifying enzyme ability of 110 patients with breast cancer with that of 113 women not affected by breast cancer. They found that abnormal glutathione-S-transferase genes resulted in up to a fourfold increased risk of breast cancer. This is a critically important finding, since one of the genetic variants of this gene is found to occur in 45 to 50 percent of the population and has also been shown to cause an increased risk of smoking-related lung cancer. In fact, Regina Santella, Ph.D., associate professor in the Division of Environmental Sciences at Columbia University in New York, stated in a 1994 interview with *Oncology Times* that "it also appears that the protective effect for vitamin E is more important in people who are missing . . . a gene for glutathione-S-transferase M1, an enzyme that can detoxify or conjugate the reactive metabolites of aromatic hydrocarbons," such as those in cigarette smoke.

Dr. Santella has developed an assay (test) that can detect early molecular damage known to be the first step in lung cancer development. These warning signs, called DNA adducts, occur three times as often in smokers than in nonsmokers. She has found that vitamin E can protect against this damage. Since vitamin E can increase the levels of glutathione-S-transferase via a portion of the DNA called the antioxidant responsive element (ARE), this may explain her findings.

I'd like to suggest some of the things you can do to increase your levels of glutathione and thus optimize the functioning of Phase 2 enzymes. Let's first consider where glutathione comes from.

Some of it, although not as much as we need, is obtained directly from such fruits and vegetables as grapefruit, oranges, strawberries, tomatoes, melons (including cantaloupe and watermelon), potatoes, broccoli, spinach, parsley, acorn squash and zucchini, asparagus, and avocado. Much more glutathione, however, gets created from the amino acids released in the breakdown of protein foods. (Indeed, many amino acids are themselves used in the Phase 2 detoxification process.)

One of the best sources of glutathione is N-acetyl-cysteine. This stable form of the amino acid L-cysteine is well tolerated, well absorbed, and easily converted to glutathione when taken supplementally. This can be important for people who aren't getting enough glutathione to keep their Phase 2 system functioning up to par. Glutathione itself in tablet form is very hard to absorb. If a physician knowledgeable about nutrition believes your detoxification system is not being adequately nourished, N-acetyl-cysteine supplements might be advisable.

A number of foods and nutrients stimulate the entire process of Phase 2 activity. Broccoli and spinach are good detoxification promoters. All members of the cruciferous vegetable family contain indoles that help push Phase 2. D-limonene, a phytonutrient from the rind of the bitter orange, is possibly the strongest Phase 2 promoter. Green tea and turmeric, the yellowish brown pigment in curry, also flood the liver with antioxidants and thereby help detoxification. These foods promote Phase 2 by direct effects on the genes—predominantly in the liver but also in the lungs and the intestinal tract—that are coded to stimulate this enzymatic activity. The chemical products of these foods actually bind to specific areas of DNA.

Certain other substances support the detoxification game plan. The recent news about broccoli sprouts' preventing cancer because of their extremely high concentration of sulforaphane (see Chapter 9) reminds me that sulforaphane is also a chemical agent that very actively promotes liver detoxification. The ellagic acid found in strawberries, raspberries, grapes, black currants, and walnuts have a very interesting role to play in detoxification as well. They have been shown to stimulate the Phase 2 enzymes while modulating the activity of Phase 1 enzymes. The physicians and nutritionists of the future will be able to tell you whether your Phase 1 enzymes seem to be running too far ahead of your Phase 2 enzymes in the total detoxification process. For now, however, it's good to know that the whole process can be fine-tuned by consuming the right phytonutrients.

Two final nutrients are well worth mentioning because they increase the efficiency of glutathione.

Silymarin is the isoflavonoid found in the milk thistle plant (see Chapter 10). It is a powerful antioxidant and seems to be particularly effective in the liver. In fact, it protects liver cells from toxic damage and, in the process, supports glutathione levels indirectly by minimizing the amount—yes, of glutathione—that is consumed in an antioxidant role.

Selenium is another important antioxidant mineral that acts as a co-factor with glutathione. It interacts with an enzyme, glutathione peroxidase, that actually speeds up glutathione's neutralization of free radicals, thereby giving you more bang for your buck.

It may seem astonishing that so many substances can play a role in supporting detoxification, but this is the way the body works. It is far from accidental that most people who eat an extraordinarily varied, nutrient-rich diet are extraordinarily healthy people.

A SELECTION OF STUDIES

There is an almost alarming multitude of studies demonstrating the effectiveness of glutathione and its most notable amino acid helpmate, N-acetyl-cysteine (NAC). I will mention just two to give you an idea of what the scientific community is now discovering.

A study done on 50 patients with advanced gastric cancer who were being treated with chemotherapy found that glutathione administration significantly decreased the toxicity of the chemotherapy without in any way diminishing its effectiveness.

Scientists have found that elderly people with higher levels of glutathione perceived themselves as healthier and, in fact, were healthier. They had fewer illnesses, lower cholesterol levels, lower blood pressure, and less body fat with more muscle.

You and your liver are lifelong allies in the war against cancer. As you begin to practice a phytonutrient-rich eating plan, know this: you will be taking some of the pressure off your liver, that ever necessary, hardworking organ. This can have only favorable results for your total health.

CHAPTER 5

NUTRIENT ANTIOXIDANTS

I don't want to attain immortality through my work, I want to attain immortality through not dying.

—WOODY ALLEN

The bright green world of the phytonutrients and antioxidants is the heart and soul of a cancer prevention program, no doubt about that. In half the chapters in this book, I will be discussing foods, compounds, enzymes, nutrients, vitamins, and minerals that have antioxidant activity in the body. Most of them have other beneficial functions as well. I'll explain those functions, of course, but don't discount their plain old fashioned antioxidant virtues. A good antioxidant is the purest coin of the realm, for those metabolic nasties, the free radicals, are always after you. *En garde!*

Let's consider the full range of the antioxidant protectors, since so much of this book will be devoted to them.

First, of course, there are the vitamins that we all learned about in seventh-grade science class. A few years back, a study published in *Nutrition Reviews* examined the antioxidant literature and reported that 120 of 130 studies document the protective effects of vitamins C and E and beta carotene in a variety of human cancers. That is as one would expect.

A wealth of antioxidants and phytonutrients that may be even more protective than the basic vitamins and minerals, however, are assembled around you in your local grocery store. These are the other antioxidants, the ones that aren't very often talked about in newspaper or news magazine articles, but they may be almost as important as the others for protecting you. This cancer answer, then, is heaped up on your fresh-food shelves. Rather than waiting for a cancer cure to be found in some high-tech lab, why not turn to nature's chemicals for a high dose of cancer prevention? In a sense, the food you see on your produce shelves is nothing but bags of chemicals that Mother Nature has manufactured for your delight in widely varying colors, flavors, sizes, and shapes.

Many of these chemicals undoubtedly still wait to be identified, but many of the most potent anticancer compounds in Mother Nature's pharmaceutical chest have already been isolated and described. Look at the food breakdown below.

PHYTONUTRIENTS AND ANTIOXIDANTS FOUND IN FOODS

Onions:
Methyl propyldisulfide
Dipropyl tetrasulfide
1-Propenyl methyl disulfide
Methyl 3,4-dimethyl-2 thienyl
    disulfide

Cabbage:
Allyl isothiocyanate
3-methylsulfinylpropyl
    isothiocyanate
4-methylthiobutyl isothiocyanate
2-phenylethyl isothiocyanate
Benzyl isothiocyanate
Chlorophyllin

Broccoli:
Indole-3 carbinol (I3C)
Allyl isothiocyanate
3-butenyl isothiocyanate
Glutamine
Chlorophyllin

Tea:
Catechin
Epicatechin
Epigallocatechin
Epigallocatechin-3-gallate (EGCG)
Tanins
Quercetin

Celery:
Psoralen
Methoxsalen
Beyapten
Trioxsalen

Oranges:
Limonene
Pinane
Limonin
Numilin
Isolimonic acid

Tomatoes:
Lycopene
Isocoumarin
Lutein
Zeaxanthin

Algae:
Chlorophyllin
Quercetin
Cryptoxanthin

Grapes:
Ellagic acid
Ellagitannin
Proanthocyandin (O.P.C.)
N-propyl gallate
Resveritol

Sesame seeds / oil:
Sesamolinol
Pinoresinol
Tocopherol
Sesamol

Those names represent a battalion of phytonutrients and antioxidants that would make any cancer tremble. Believe me, you need them. The free-radical theory of disease causation is well accepted today. We know that those fiendishly active and thoroughly unbalanced molecules are a chief contributor to many of the most exceptionally devastating diseases, including heart disease and cancer. You are the dartboard into which trillions of free-radical reactions hurl their energy daily. If you didn't have formidable defenses, you would soon be just another set of trophy antlers hanging in the den of the free-radical empire!

Fortunately, you are well equipped. You can turn to the natural-food packages that we've just described. You can go even further and add supplements. I always emphasize natural antioxidants—foods—first. Nature does know what she's doing, and just as you can stay alive and full of energy by eating food, so you can place a zillion roadblocks in front of cancer. That, after all, is what a clove of garlic or a head of cabbage or a cup of green tea is—a formidable natural roadblock that an enterprising young cancer cell will have a difficult time getting around.

Nonetheless, you can't be too well protected in a land where one of every three people eventually winds up hearing the words "You have cancer." In the final balance, I come down in favor of vigorous protection. That means that supplementation with a number of nutrients, herbs, enzymes, vitamins, and minerals is advisable. In this chapter, we're going to look at a number of exceptionally interesting nutritional antioxidants just so you can get your feet wet. All of them have applications for cancer, but in many cases, we'll pause and make a deep bow in the direction of their ability to protect you from cardiovascular ills and many other dreadful fates.

PYCNOGENOL® AND GRAPE SEED EXTRACT

In 1534, French explorer Jacques Cartier, got himself frozen in on the St. Lawrence River in Canada. His situation was dire. On board his ship, he carried only biscuits and frozen meat. He and his men would have died from scurvy on such a diet long before spring arrived. Luckily, the Frenchmen were rescued by the local Indians, who showed them how to brew a tea from the needles and bark of the *anneda* pine tree. The beverage contained minute quantities of vitamin C and very considerable quantities of a bioflavonoid that has since been dubbed Pycnogenol.

From that time until almost the present, no one gave much thought to the brew that saved Cartier. Then in the 1950s, Professor Jacques Masqueliler of the University of Bordeaux in France perfected a method of extracting certain plant flavonoids called proanthocyanidins from pine bark. He dubbed these active components Pycnogenol, patented them, and then in the 1970s began working on very similar proanthocyanidins taken from grape seeds. Most of what follows applies to both Pycnogenol and grape seed extract, although I will generally refer to Pycnogenol, the better-known and more frequently discussed substance. Keep in mind, however, that some researchers now regard grape seed extract as an effective preparation.

These proanthocyanidins are among the most powerful antioxidants ever discovered. Tests have shown that Pycnogenol is 20 times more powerful than vitamin C and 50 times more powerful than vitamin E as a free-radical scavenger. Researchers demonstrated that Pycnogenol vigorously went after such classic oxidant bad guys as superoxide, hydroxyl, and peroxide radicals. Pycnogenol is water soluble, meaning that it dissolves in water and moves freely through your bloodstream. (Fat-soluble nutrients, on the other hand, dissolve only in fat, entering thereby into your tissues.)

Pharmacist's Corner

■ **Pycnogenol®**: a pine bark extract supplying active ingredients known as OPC's. Take from 25 to 100 milligrams daily with a glass of juice or water.

■ Pycnogenol supports blood vessel walls and connective tissue in the skin.

This nontoxic bioflavonoid has become a best-selling nutritional supplement in Europe, but it is still overlooked in America except by the cognoscenti. Pycnogenol and grape seed extract are no longer experimental, however, and certainly not of dubious efficacy. Proanthocyandins have been shown to lower cholesterol levels and to reduce the size of arterial cholesterol deposits in humans and animals. Minor vascular problems also seem amenable to pycnogenol. A German study that gave patients with varicose veins 90 milligrams of pycnogenol daily found that 77 percent improved significantly. Diabetic retinopathy also appears to respond.

One of Pycnogenol's most interesting effects is on collagen, the major structural protein that holds together the cells and tissues of the body. Collagen is degraded by age and the collapsing of the cross-linkages of collagen fibers that give them strength. That's one

---

Different Amounts for Different People?

Do you get enough of the major beneficial nutrients? The amounts of each that you need depend on your lifestyle, your genetics, your absorptive capacities, and your physical environment. Smokers, for instance, deplete the body's store of antioxidants. What is worse, there is a detoxification enzyme called glutathione-s-transferase that breaks down carcinogens, such as the benzoprene found in cigarette smoke, and this enzyme is deficient in a significant percent of the population. It has been shown that smokers whose genes predispose them to lower levels of glutathione-S-transferase are at an increased risk of lung cancer. It has also been shown by researchers at the Columbia University School of Public Health in New York that individuals who had sufficiently high levels of vitamin E received considerable protection even if their levels of glutathione-S-transferase were low.

Dr. Bruce Ames, an internationally known scientist who invented the Ames test for measuring the carcinogenic potential of chemicals, has suggested that it would be useful for physicians to routinely assay levels of vitamins. "With these assays," Dr. Ames noted, "physicians quickly could determine whether patients have sufficient levels of folic acid, ascorbate, vitamin E, and other beneficial nutrients." At the Strang Cancer Prevention Center in New York, it is now a policy to monitor vitamin levels to determine how much supplementation is needed. I believe an increasing number of major cancer centers around the country will soon learn to do this.

of the reasons your skin sags as you get older. Pycnogenol appears to be the most effective substance for maintaining the integrity of collagen yet discovered.

Meanwhile, there have been indications that Pycnogenol® is no friend to cancer, which is not surprising for an antioxidant of its strength. Stewart Brown, Ph.D., of the University of Nottingham in England, reported, at an international symposium on Pycnogenol, that the proanthocyanidins free-radical scavenging slows the mutation of cancer cells. At the same symposium, D. White, Ph.D., announced that Pycnogenol inhibits the creation of one of the most significant carcinogens in tobacco smoke, the highly destructive diole epoxide of benzoprene.

Since drinking pine bark tea, or even chewing the stuff, is not an appetizing alternative, Pycnogenol is one substance that I recommend you take in supplemental form just like a daily multivitamin. In Europe, millions of people have been taking this bioflavonoid since the 1960s, and it appears to be as safe as it is potent and attractive.

LIPOIC ACID

Lipoic acid is a substance that the human body creates internally and obtains from food. In fact, it appears to be an essential component of the system our body uses to unlock energy from food. Scientists believe that lipoic acid directs food into energy production and away from fat production. In addition, lipoic acid is an almost unique antioxidant and a powerful detoxifier of heavy metals.

There appears to be a problem with this compound, however: namely, supply. The body makes barely enough for its metabolic needs, and age, disease, and environmental conditions can cause outright deficiency. Even under the best of circumstances, it seems unlikely that we produce enough lipoic acid for it to carry out its antioxidant functions in an optimal manner. It's possible to redress the imbalance through food and supplementation.

Lipoic acid's remarkable activity as an antioxidant is centered around its ability to be soluble in both water-based and fat-based compartments of the body. Virtually all other antioxidants have

Pharmacist's Corner

■ **Lipoic acid** is also referred to as alpha-lipoic acid and it is found in small quantities in red meat and yeast.

■ **Lipoic acid:** take 30 milligrams to 100 milligrams daily with a meal.

■ Studies indicate that higher dosage levels are helpful with diabetes-related peripheral neuropathy. This dosage ranges from a minimum of 300 milligrams to a maximum of 900 milligrams daily, according to a number of studies.

■ **Lipoic acid** has a short half-life, meaning that it lasts for only a very short time in our system and is excreted quickly from our bodies. Therefore, it is helpful to split the daily dosage into two or three parts.

their primary activity in either water or fat—not both. Vitamin C, for instance, is essentially water soluble. Vitamin E is essentially fat soluble. Lipoic acid is the versatile antioxidant.

Moreover, it appears capable of regenerating some of the other antioxidants, particularly vitamin E. Cardiovascular studies have repeatedly shown that vitamin E is the primary antioxidant protecting cholesterol from free-radical damage—that is, from oxidation. Most people have a negative impression of cholesterol, but it is actually one of the most vital substances in your body, essential for the building of your cell walls and your nerve sheaths. It's only when cholesterol is attacked by free radicals that it becomes damaging to your arteries. Vitamin E protects it from oxidation but can itself be consumed by free radicals unless the vitamin is recycled back into its undamaged form by supporting antioxidants like lipoic acid. Lipoic acid also recycles vitamin C quite effectively.

There can be no doubt that the powerful antioxidant effects of lipoic acid are themselves cancer preventive. Richard Passwater, Ph.D., a prominent antioxidant researcher for many decades, has also suggested that the compound can do more than that. He believes that lipoic acid prevents nuclear factor kappa-B (NF kappa-

B) from activating oncogenes, the genes that cause cancer when they are acted on by a carcinogen. According to Passwater, "Dietary lipoic acid can enter the cytosol of cells and protect NF kappa-B from activation by radiation, free radicals, or even sunlight."

Certainly, lipoic acid deserves to receive some of the intensive research that has been lavished on other antioxidants since the 1980s.

COENZYME CoQ$_{10}$

If I were writing a book on heart disease instead of cancer, I could really go to town on coenzyme CoQ$_{10}$. This is a fabulous nutrient so widespread throughout the body that it is also called by the name ubiquinone, as in *ubiquitous*. It is most concentrated in the heart, and various clinical trials have demonstrated that people with heart disease who take CoQ$_{10}$ have increased survival rates and improvements in their quality of life. CoQ$_{10}$ acts as a catalyst in the mitochondria, the energy factories of our cells, for the generation of ATP (adenosine triphosphate), one of the main forms of energy in the human body. There are reports from many sources that CoQ$_{10}$ increases exercise capacity as well.

CoQ$_{10}$ has many positive qualities, such as being a vigorous antioxidant, and some researchers believe that the existence of a cancer correlates strongly with reduced levels of this compound. Researchers at the University of Texas, encouraged by the positive indications of CoQ$_{10}$'s effect on immune function, gave it to seven patients with acquired immunodeficiency syndrome (AIDS) a few years ago and noticed major improvements in five of them.

The bad news in the midst of all this nutritional good news is that levels of CoQ$_{10}$ begin declining as we age. No one knows at what point this decline becomes serious, but the arguments for supplementing CoQ$_{10}$ by the time we reach our forties or fifties are strong ones.

From a strict cancer perspective, doctors are waiting with intense interest to see if further studies confirm the results obtained in Copenhagen, Denmark, when 32 high-risk patients with breast cancer were given 90 micrograms of CoQ$_{10}$ a day by Knud Lock-

---

Pharmacist's Corner

■ **Coenzyme CoQ$_{10}$:** take 30 milligrams to 100 milligrams daily with food.

■ Patients with heart disease and those with poorly functioning immune systems are often advised to take 100 milligrams three times a day with food.

■ Manufacturers of an emulsified version claim that it is three times more absorbable than the classic form of CoQ$_{10}$; therefore, a 30-milligram version of the emulsified form should supply as much CoQ$_{10}$ as a 90-milligram version of the common form. More studies need to be performed to prove this point.

■ **Possible drug interaction:** There is a report that CoQ$_{10}$ may decrease the effectiveness of the anticoagulant drug warfarin, (Coumadin). If you are on this blood thinner, do not start taking CoQ$_{10}$ without informing your doctor. If you are already on CoQ$_{10}$ while taking warfarin, do not stop taking it without informing your doctor.

---

wood, M.D., a breast cancer specialist. After several months of treatment, there was partial tumor remission in six of the women and, after two years, all of the original subjects of the study were still alive, although at least four deaths would normally have been expected.

More startling still were two cases involving women for whom the dosage was increased to more than 300 milligrams a day. In both the women, the tumor shrank until it was no longer palpable and could not be found by mammography. By that point, both women were in excellent health. Dr. Lockwood, who has treated about 200 patients with breast cancer a year for 35 years, reported that he had never before seen "a spontaneous complete regression of a 1.5- to 2.0-centimeter breast tumor."

Clearly, we are just at the beginning of CoQ$_{10}$ cancer research. This is a nontoxic antioxidant with multiple health advantages, however, and I believe a modest level of supplementation, perhaps 30 milligrams a day, would be advisable for people who are middle-aged or older. Women who are at high risk for breast cancer should consult their doctors about the possibility of taking a higher dose. CoQ_{10} is oil soluble, so it should be taken with meals and thus absorbed together with the fat in your food.

RESVERATROL

In the early 1990s, people began to speak about the "French paradox.": the intriguing fact that the French consume at least as much fat as Americans, smoke more cigarettes, and yet have a heart disease rate that's less than 50 percent of ours. It didn't seem fair. A lot of thought was given to explaining it. One of the most cogent explanations scientists came up with was France's high national consumption of wine.

As it happens, wine—especially red wine—is packed with a bunch of phytonutrient compounds, such as tannins, phenols, and epicatechins, that may sound unalluring to your ears but that are mighty effective antioxidants. They tend to reduce blood clotting, as well as having other effects that would plausibly lead to the reduction of heart disease.

One of these health-enhancing substances is called resveratrol, and new research has shown it to be a powerful cancer-fighting agent as well. Resveratrol turns up in many foods, but it occurs in high concentrations only in red grapes and peanuts. Peanuts I can't recommend to you, since they have a less than ideal level of fatty acids and occasionally contain traces of a potent carcinogen called aflatoxin. (Rumor has it that highly concentrated aflatoxin was one of the chemical agents Saddam Hussein used on American troops in 1991 during Operation Desert Storm during the Persian Gulf War. Red grapes, however, I heartily recommend—especially those that come from regions that are cold and damp, such as France and Canada. As a rule, such grapes (and the wines made from them) have much higher concentrations of resveratrol than grapes and wines from warmer climates, say, in California, Italy, Spain, or Portugal.

Resveratrol is a phenol that vigorously inhibits our old nemesis the cyclooxygenase-2 (COX-2) enzyme, the promoter of inflammation and ultimately cancer. It also does good things for the wine itself through its potent antifungal activity. It has been shown in experiments that resveratrol can block the oxidation of low-density lipoprotein (LDL) cholesterol, sometimes called "bad" cholesterol, one of the major causes of atherosclerosis.

For our purposes, the significance of this grape-derived phyto-nutrient lies in its recently demonstrated effects on cancer. In 1997, scientists at the University of Illinois in Urbana-Champaign published a study on the effect of resveratrol on mice with skin cancer tumors. In the mice given the highest dose, the number of tumors was reduced by 98 percent compared with untreated mice, and the number of mice who developed tumors at all dropped by 88 percent in that group. This is a good starting point for further research.

Scientists at Ohio State University College of Medicine and Public Health reported that a diet rich in black raspberries prevented chemically induced esophageal cancers in rats. This study was presented in 1998 in New Orleans at the annual meeting of the American Association for Cancer Research. The number of tumors fell appreciably in rats fed the black raspberry diet. Black raspberries are high in a chemical similar to resveratrol called ellagic acid.

Pharmacist's Corner

■ Resveratrol is most concentrated in red wines from cold regions, such as French Cabernets, but since resveratrol lasts for just a very short time in the body, healthy men may consider drinking a glass of red wine with lunch and dinner.

■ Once a wine bottle is opened, its resveratrol evaporates within 1 day at room temperature, but if the bottle is refrigerated, the resveratrol will last for about 1 week.

■ Because there is strong evidence that drinking alcohol causes breast cancer, women should minimize alcohol intake. Women are better off taking a 1,000-microgram resveratrol capsule once or twice a day with a small glass of grape juice.

When it comes to the resveratrol story, the bottom line is that grapes and similar products are capable of reducing your risk for heart disease and perhaps cancer as well. The interesting question is in what form you should obtain them. Considerable research in the 1990s has demonstrated rather convincingly that a moderate consumption of alcohol—one to two drinks a day—is, in fact, health enhancing, principally because of its effects on blood cholesterol levels. Red wine has additional health-enhancing phytonutrients, one of which is resveratrol. If there was no such thing as immoderation in drinking, I would unhesitatingly suggest that you consume a glass of red wine daily. As it is, I think you should do so only if you are thoroughly convinced that you and your blood relatives have no history of drinking problems.

Those of you who would rather not take up wine drinking can still obtain small quantities of resveratrol by drinking dark grape juice and eating red grapes. It's not a bad way of protecting your health.

WHY BUGS BUNNY LOOKS SO YOUNG: CAROTENOIDS

Natural forces are the healers of disease.

—HIPPOCRATES

Bugs Bunny, that carrot-chewing rabbit, certainly knew how to keep his hop! He consumed large amounts of carotenoids. The carotenoids are a group of fat-soluble pigments found in orange, red, yellow, and dark green vegetables and fruits—that is, in foods ranging from carrots, tomatoes, squash, watermelon, pink grapefruit, and sweet potatoes to spinach, kale, lettuce, and brussels sprouts. Chemical relatives of vitamin A, carotenoids are the most common pigments in nature and produce a red and orange coloration, though, in the case of the green plants, the color of chlorophyll hides the pigmentation. There are over 600 carotenoids that have been isolated from plant foods. About 50 of them have some ability to convert to vitamin A in our livers, and 50 to 60 of them are consumed in a typical diet. Of course, there may be—and probably are—many, many more we know nothing about.

Science is in the early stages of untangling the carotenoid story. It's a thriller. Everything we know so far seems to show that carotenoids are nearly as vital for life as the essential vitamins and minerals; yet, we are only clumsily beginning to figure out which carotenoids do what. That's why this chapter—even more than many others in this book—is a report in progress. Nonetheless, what we know right now gives us confidence. If you live a normal lifetime without ever encountering cancer, then one of the main reasons for your immunity will be the protection these special nutritional pigments gave you.

All members of the carotenoid family are related in chemical structure to vitamin A, the most important vitamin for immune function. Indeed, beta carotene, the carotenoid that almost everyone has heard of, is sometimes referred to as provitamin A because the body is capable of partially converting it into vitamin A; of all the carotenoids, it has the greatest ability to perform this conversion. This was originally considered to be beta carotene's most important characteristic. Vitamin A, the first vitamin ever discovered, is a powerhouse nutrient that stimulates the immune system, fights infections, and maintains the structural integrity of cells by allowing their genetic material to split properly.

Most of us can get our primary supplies of vitamin A from beta carotene conversion, which is convenient and safe because excess quantities of A are toxic, whereas beta carotene virtually never is. Sometimes people with hypothyroidism or diabetes will have difficulty converting beta carotene to vitamin A; they must be sure to get sufficient vitamin A through their diet or by supplementation.

Time has shown that beta carotene has many other excellent properties in addition to its chemical convertibility to vitamin A. It is an antioxidant in its own right and stimulates T-helper cells in the immune system, the cells so important to ridding the body of invaders.

It is believed, however, that the most significant characteristic of beta carotene is its association with lowered cancer risk. Studies have repeatedly shown that a higher dietary intake of beta carotene is associated with a diminished likelihood of several cancers, particularly lung, stomach, and breast cancer. Of course, a high intake of beta carotene inevitably means a high intake of many other carotenoids. Scientists are currently only guessing at whether beta carotene or its helpmates play a greater role here.

In fact, scientists have already learned that many of the other carotenoids have even greater antioxidant activity than does beta carotene. This includes such newly discovered nutritional heavyweights as alpha- and gamma-carotene, lycopene, canthaxanthin, lutein, and zeaxanthin. I think we should take a look at a few of these carotenoids individually before returning to consider the entire carotenoid team, the cozy nutritional collective that may be one of the major reasons you're cancer free.

One note of caution—the new fat substitute Olestra, found in certain snack foods, can reduce blood levels of carotenoids by 50 percent by inhibiting their absorption. This "antinutrient" can also interfere with the absorption of fat-soluble vitamins A, D, E, and K. I forbid my patients to consume Olestra.

LYCOPENE

Lycopene is the hot new star among the carotenoids. It's the red pigment found in tomatoes, carrots, apricots, paprika, pink grapefruit, and watermelon. For instance, a study done in 1997 on 1,379 European men indicated that those who consumed the most lycopene in their diet were half as likely to suffer a heart attack as those who consumed the least.

I didn't need to know that to be excited about lycopene, for it seems to be one of the most powerful antioxidants in the human diet and a vigilant cancer fighter. Researchers have demonstrated that overall, it exhibits the highest rate of all carotenoids for quenching singlet oxygen, a particularly virulent form of free radical. Few people are aware that lycopene's anti–free radical activity is roughly double that of beta carotene. This almost certainly has some role in its well-attested capacity to lower levels of breast, lung, endometrial, cervical, and prostate cancers and cancers of the digestive tract—from mouth to anus.

Some of the most enticing lycopene evidence relates to the prostate. Specifically, your prostate loves tomatoes. Scientists conducting the huge Health Professionals Follow-up Study with 47,000 subjects found that reduced levels of prostate cancer were dramatically associated with higher levels of lycopene consumption and that 82 percent of that lycopene was drawn from the combined intake of tomatoes, tomato paste, tomato sauce, tomato juice, and pizza. At the higher levels of this consumption, it was found that a man who eats 10 servings of tomato-based foods per week reduces his prostate cancer risk by 45 percent!

Nutritionists usually advise us to eat fresh fruits and vegetables and eat them raw when possible. Good advice, for the most part; but in the case of lycopene and tomatoes, we know that cooked is better—and processed is better yet. The digestive system can extract only a limited amount of lycopene from fresh tomatoes because the pigmented carotenoid is locked in a matrix of proteins and fiber. Cooking breaks down the cell walls and frees the carotenoid. If you don't like cooked tomatoes, your best bet for getting a prostate-saving dose of lycopene is to eat plenty of tomato paste and sauce with your meals—and even ketchup, which is, in other respects, anything but a healthy food. The fat in these processed foods also permits better absorption of lycopene.

Further research has shown that lycopene protects against cancer of the mouth, pharynx, esophagus, stomach, colon, and rectum. Moreover, Israeli studies conducted on breast, lung, and endome-

Lycopene Levels in Foods

Lycopene is found in relatively few foods. Here are the main sources, measured as milligrams of lycopene per 100 grams (100 grams is approximately 3⅓ ounces).

Source	Milligrams per 100 Grams
Apricot, canned	0.06
Apricot, dried	0.80
Grapefruit, pink and raw	3.40
Guava juice	3.30
Tomato, raw	3.10
Tomato juice, canned	8.60
Tomato paste, canned	6.50
Tomato sauce, canned	6.30
Watermelon, raw	4.10

From Mangels A. R., et al., "Carotenoid content of fruits and vegetables: an evaluation of analytic data," *Journal of the American Dietetic Association,* 1993;93:284–286, with permission.

trial cancer cell cultures showed that lycopene inhibited the growth of those cells, basically by slowing the rate of their division. All this accords very well with the conclusions of one research group that reported a 50 percent reduction in the rate for cancers of all sites among elderly Americans with a high tomato intake.

Of course, men with prostate troubles are the first people I send to the tomato patch. Tom Grimaud, a 50-year-old attorney, was sent to me for nutritional advice because his prostate gland was mildly enlarged and his level of prostate-specific antigen (PSA), detected in a screening test, was about twice as high as it ought to be. A biopsy had revealed that there were abnormal cells in his prostate, but fortunately there was no evidence that they had become cancerous yet. I told Tom to take vitamin E because I knew of a recent study that demonstrated that the vitamin sharply reduces the rate of prostate cancer. I also encouraged him to eat lots of green peas, baked beans, and garlic because there has been solid research relating all of these to reduced risk of prostate cancer. Finally, I would have liked to tell him to eat tomatoes daily, but he had a lifelong aversion to the vegetable. Instead, I told him to take lycopene supplements. When Tom saw his urologist six months later, his PSA had gone down by 25 percent and another prostate biopsy revealed that no evidence existed of abnormal or premalignant lesions. I think Tom now has a solid phytonutrient defense team working for him.

LUTEIN AND ZEAXANTHIN

Lutein and zeaxanthin, two carotenoids heavily present in kale, collard greens, spinach, corn, yellow squash, and most other yellow fruits and veggies, are associated with decreased breast cancer risk. It's not known yet if they protect against other cancers as well, but considering the foods they're found in, it would be surprising if they did not.

Researchers have demonstrated that these carotenoids help protect the eyes from macular degeneration, the main cause of blindness in older people. Lutein especially is found in very high concentrations in the macula, the part of the retina that distinguishes fine detail at the center of the field of vision.

ALL TOGETHER

It may well be that teamwork is best. As you're already beginning to notice, the emphasis of this book is on the maximum intake of the widest variety of fruits and vegetables for cancer protection. Here are a few studies that indicate the combined effect of carotenoids on cancer risk:

- A 1997 study in Honolulu found that 69 Japanese American men with three forms of mouth and throat cancer had significantly lower blood levels of alpha carotene, beta carotene, beta-cryptoxanthin, total carotenoids, and vitamin E when compared with matched study subjects who did not have these cancers.
- In a 1996 study of 235 women in New York City reported in the *Journal of Clinical Cancer Research,* those who had cervical cancer or who showed cellular changes in the cervix that

put them at high risk for such cancer had much lower plasma levels of beta carotene, lycopene, and canthaxanthin.

- Another cervical cancer study that monitored 15,161 women for 15 years found a significant reduction in risk among women with a high level of canthaxanthin.
- A 1995 study of premenopausal breast cancer in two counties in western New York found that there was decreased breast cancer risk for women who had high levels of vegetable consumption and also specific reductions of risk associated with higher intake of alpha and beta carotene and lutein and zeaxanthin.
- It has also been observed that women who eat a carotenoid-rich diet and are later diagnosed with breast cancer have improved prospects of survival. A 1996 Michigan study found that among patients with breast cancer, those whose tumors contained estrogen receptors (which is associated with higher survival rates) had significantly higher carotenoid intake.

To some extent, all these studies indicate why beta carotene in particular has been so strongly associated with reduced cancer risk. It is the carotenoid that is most widely distributed in fruits and vegetables, and this means that blood levels of it are perhaps the best available biomarker of the consumption of such foods. Thus, beta carotene levels become a rough indicator for the entire carotenoid family, which may include not only the cancer-preventive substances we've talked about so far but also many carotenoids that haven't yet been named, discovered, researched, or understood. The study from Finland several years ago that showed, for our purposes, a contradictory result—a higher level of lung cancer in smokers taking beta carotene supplements—suggests several things. First, don't expect a few years of consuming any single nutrient to undo decades of a bad habit like smoking. Second, consumption of a mixture of carotenoids like that provided by nature is likely to be far more beneficial than consumption of a single one.

WHY DO CAROTENOIDS STOP CANCER?

Of course, we may not yet know all the reasons why these potent pigments are so protective, but scientists think they know a few.

The most obvious aspect of their potency is antioxidant protection. The cellular damage caused by free radicals easily leads to an increased rate of mutation within cells and greater risk for cancer. Research seems to show that carotenoids taken in combination defend against uncontrolled oxidation even more vigorously than such rightly heralded vitamins as A, C, and E! This doesn't mean you should ignore those other well-recognized antioxidants. They all work better as a team. And as a team, they strengthen each other synergistically, which is probably essential for the enjoyment of optimal health.

Other research suggests that carotenoids help to maintain cell differentiation. Healthy cells in the body become differentiated to perform particular tasks. They may be muscle cells or digestive tract cells or skin cells. It is a characteristic of cancer that the cells that make it up lose differentiation and become useless for any purpose except the deadly one they have evolved to perform.

Another theory is that carotenoids help promote the activities of detoxification enzymes. Whatever the truth, carotenoids are cancer fighters extraordinaire.

CAROTENOIDS AND SOME OF THE FRUITS AND VEGETABLES IN WHICH THEY'RE FOUND

Alpha and beta carotene:
Carrots
Sweet potatoes
Pumpkin
Winter squash
Yams
Cantaloupe
Beans
Broccoli
Brussels sprouts
Spinach

Cryptoxanthin:
Oranges
Grapes
Lemons

Tangerines
Apples
Corn
Poultry

Zeaxanthin:
Peaches
Corn

Canthaxanthin:
Trout
Crustaceans
Mushrooms

Lutein:
Kale
Spinach

Pharmacist's Corner

■ Carotenoids concentrate in many tissues. Some carotenoids are more important in some tissues because of this ability to concentrate. Also, many carotenoids are stronger antioxidants than beta carotene is. For these reasons, you should take a mixed carotenoid rather than just beta carotene if you are going to supplement. An example of a good mixed carotenoid supplement is the following:

Beta carotene	5,000 or more international units
Alpha carotene	1–3 milligrams
Gamma carotene	1 milligram
Lycopene	5 or more milligrams
Lutein	6 or more milligrams
Zeaxanthin	0.6 milligram or more
Cryptoxanthin	1 milligram or more

■ You can obtain all these carotenoids and more if you consume the following cross-section of vegetables daily: corn or yellow squash; spinach or broccoli; carrots; tomato products, including tomato sauce, paste, or juice; mushrooms; and plankton. Consider using some of these ingredients the next time you make fresh vegetable juice.

■ **Drug interaction:** Methotrexate, a drug used commonly in cancer chemotherapy, severe rheumatoid arthritis, and psoriasis, decreases the absorption of beta carotene. It is not known yet whether it decreases the absorption of other protective carotenoids. Patients taking methotrexate should ask their clinician if they should supplement with a mixed carotenoid containing beta carotene.

■ **Nutrient–nutrient interaction:** High-dose beta carotene supplementation can cause depletion of vitamin E in the blood, and if your doctor prescribes long-term beta carotene supplementation at doses exceeding 25,000 international units daily, you should take a vitamin E supplement.

■ Beta carotene increases the amount of liver damage caused by massive amounts of alcohol in animal studies. Because performing human studies would be unethical and because there is no guide as to what level of alcohol will interact with beta carotene, both alcoholics and people consuming more than three alcoholic beverages daily should not supplement with beta carotene. (What they should really do is cut down on the alcohol, but alas, this is not always the case.)

■ **Warning:** In both the CARET Trial, conducted by the National Cancer Institute (a division of the National Institute of Health in Bethesda, Maryland), and a large Finnish study, beta carotene increased the incidence of lung cancer in smokers, and smokers should therefore never take beta carotene as a supplement. On the other hand, beta carotene decreases the incidence of lung cancer in nonsmokers.

CHAPTER 7

OMEGA-3 OILS AND OTHER FATS

*In treating a patient, let your first thought
be to strengthen his [or her] natural
vitality.*

—RHAZES

Does a high-fat diet cause cancer? Will a fishy diet prevent malignancies? Will olive oil help? Will trans fatty acids hurt? What do all these names mean? What kind of fats are they? What is a reasonable approach to fats?

These are all pretty sensible questions, and fat, I'm afraid, is a fairly complicated business. Nonetheless, we'd better plunge in. Everybody eats a fairly high amount of fat in their diet, whether the diet they eat is called low fat or high fat. Fat, like carbohydrate and protein, is a major constituent of food, and the evidence from literally thousands of medical studies seems to show that the type of fat you eat—even more than the quantity—directly affects your likelihood of ever suffering most of the major forms of cancer.

GOOD FATS, BAD FATS, AND FATS IN BETWEEN

See the box on pages 82–83 for a compact breakdown of the different kinds of fats. Both saturated and polyunsaturated fats have been associated with many different kinds of cancer. In the case of polyunsaturated fat, however, this effect primarily depends on the type of polyunsaturate eaten. The polyunsaturates found in corn oil, for instance, appear to be carcinogenic, whereas the ones found in fish are extremely protective.

The other two principal types of fats—monounsaturates and trans fats—are very much opposites. Monounsaturates—especially olive oil—are extremely healthy foods when eaten in moderation. Indeed, evidence suggests that they help oppose cancer.

Trans fats (often referred to on food packaging as hydrogenated oils), on the other hand, are artificial fats not found in nature and are far from benign. The American food industry developed them

81

Overview of Fats

There are four basic kinds of fats found in our diets.

Saturated fats
Saturated fats are solid at room temperature. They are primarily found in animal products.

Food sources: whole milk; cream; cheese; butter; fatty meats, such as beef, veal, lamb, pork, and ham; vegetable products, such as coconut oil, palm kernel oil, and vegetable shortening.

The connection between saturated fats and cancer is not yet clear; however, the liver uses saturated fats to manufacture cholesterol. Therefore, people who have high cholesterol levels will need to restrict their intake.

Polyunsaturated fats
Polyunsaturates come in two forms: omega-3 and omega-6 fats.

OMEGA-3 FATTY ACIDS
Omega-3 fatty acids are found in fish, plankton, and certain vegetable products.

Food sources: cold-water fish, such as salmon, mackerel, eel, tuna, herring, halibut, cod, and sardines; flaxseed, hempseed, cattail seed, and walnut oils.

Omega-3 fatty acids appear to protect against both cardiovascular disease and cancer.

OMEGA-6 FATTY ACIDS
Omega-6 fatty acids are found in vegetable products.

Food sources: corn, cottonseed, safflower, and sunflower oils.

Omega-6 fatty acids will often lower total cholesterol levels, but in large amounts, they also have a tendency to reduce heart-protective high-density lipoprotein (HDL) cholesterol, sometimes called "good" cholesterol. They have been consistently associated with increased cancer risk.

Monosaturated fatty acids
Monounsaturated fatty acids are found in vegetable products.

Food sources: vegetable and nut oil, including olive and peanut oil; by far, the largest percentage is in olive oil.

Monosaturated fatty acids appear to protect against both cardiovascular disease and cancer.

Trans fatty acids

Trans fatty acids are not found in nature.

Food sources: These fats are inserted into margarine and most baked goods to harden liquid vegetable oil and to increase the stability and shelf life of the product.

Trans fatty acids may be a commercial bonanza, but from the point of view of health, it would be better if no one ever ate a molecule of them again. They appear to be associated with increased risk of both heart disease and cancer.

by hydrogenating vegetable oil to create margarine, in the process coming up with a substance that made baked goods firmer and less crumbly. The operation was commercially successful, to say the least, but many—if not most—scientists now think that trans fatty acids, with their twisted, unnatural molecules, are entirely unhealthy and may contribute on some level to lowering a cell's protection against cancer.

Moreover, the Harvard Nurses' Study, one of the largest, longest running, most carefully monitored studies in the history of American medicine, has provided yet another reason to run away from trans fats. In a 1993 report, the Harvard researchers found that among the 85,000 nurses in their study, those who consumed large amounts of margarine had a 66 percent greater risk of heart disease than did low consumers of margarine. That is a colossal figure. By contrast, the correlation of heart disease and butter consumption was minor. Margarine and other hydrogenated oils are a cardiovascular double whammy because they not only raise levels of harmful low-density lipoprotein (LDL) cholesterol but also lower levels of protective HDL cholesterol.

Quite clearly, therefore, choosing monosaturated fat and avoiding trans fats will be easy for you. The real decision making in your diet will revolve around the kinds of saturated and polyunsaturated fat you should be eating, as well as which you should be eating more and less of.

Because I generally stress the positive rather than the negative, I think we ought to turn our attention now to some of the healthiest fats you can put in your diet.

FINNY FRIENDS

A diet high in deep and cold-water fish (haddock, cod, salmon, tuna, halibut, mackerel, sardines) has been associated with a decreased risk of both heart disease and cancer. As far as we know, this is principally because these fish contain a type of oil called omega-3 fatty acid. This remarkable substance is concentrated in the flesh of cold-water fish because omega-3 oils don't solidify until the temperature drops to − 103° Fahrenheit. Therefore, the colder the water a fish lives in, the more omega-3 its body requires and possesses, simply to keep it warm enough. We could actually get the same excellent substance by eating polar-bear burgers or whale steaks, but since most of us don't indulge, it's probably best to stick to fish.

Omega-3 oils come in three forms. One, which we'll discuss shortly, is found in certain plants. The other two—both found in fish—are docosahexaenoic acid (DHA), essential for brain and eye development in children, and eicosapentaenoic acid (EPA), a substance whose anti-inflammatory influence seems to have a great many positive effects in the body.

One thing is certain: omega-3 oils help to protect mammals like you and me from cancer, something that has been documented repeatedly since the late 1980s in a diverse variety of human and animal studies. These oils protect us from other things as well. They have been found to be effective in reducing inflammatory processes in such conditions as psoriasis, rheumatoid arthritis, ulcerative colitis, allergies, and asthma.

Meanwhile, Bruce Ames, Ph.D., the noted cancer researcher at the University of California at Berkeley, has hypothesized that chronic inflammatory states can lead to cancer by increasing the production of free radicals, which damage deoxyribonucleic acid (DNA). Since the oils found in fish help to inhibit this inflammation, they help prevent cancer. Indeed, the lower incidence of cancer in Eskimos compared with other North Americans has been attributed to their consumption of omega-3 oil fatty acids. If Eskimos eat as much fish as they're said to eat, you shouldn't be surprised. Let's look at what the scientists have uncovered when they compare fish eaters to non–fish eaters.

Real Brain Food!

Docosahexaenoic acid (DHA) not only inhibits cancer but also is the primary structural fatty acid found in the brain—which is about 60 percent fat—and the retina of the eye. Scientists have discovered that adequate levels of DHA are essential for proper brain development during pregnancy and early childhood. The amount of DHA obtained in breast milk can be critical for a child's future intellectual development. Additional research also indicates that DHA supports optimal brain function and continued mental acuity throughout life.

There is one big study from Europe that is really an eye-opener. British scientists compared the mortality data for breast and colorectal cancer in 24 European countries. They found that cancer rates rose with increased consumption of animal fat, but cancer rates decreased when fish and fish oil consumption increased. The lower cancer rates associated with fish and fish oil consumption were statistically significant whether the intakes were measured in the current time period or 10 years before or up to 23 years before. For both men and women, the cancer rates fell when the fish consumption went up.

Another interesting piece of research was done in Finland and measured the fatty acid composition of the breast tissue in women with breast cancer and in patients with benign breast disease. The one significant difference researchers discovered was that the women who had breast cancer had much lower levels of EPA and DHA (the fatty acids in omega-3 fish oil) in their breast tissue.

Finally, a recent Japanese study showed that the risk of developing prostate cancer was higher in men who ate little or no seafood. In experimental animals as well, omega-3 fatty acids have consistently protected against tumor formation.

Balance the Prostaglandins

All the positive effects of omega-3 fatty acids are believed to be due to the fatty acids' capacity to inhibit the formation of chemicals in our bodies called prostaglandins. Certain prostaglandins, especially one called PGE-2 (prostaglandin E-2), have been associated with inflammatory states; tumor growth, including prostate, breast, and colon cancer growth; and suppression of the immune system's ability to spot tumors. I'm sure you remember the damning list of PGE-2's cancer-promoting effects that I included in Chapter 3 (see 37–38).

The fish oils containing EPA and DHA are converted to more beneficial prostaglandins called PGE-3 prostaglandins. PGE-3 has its own series of powerful effects, too, which includes inhibiting the enzymes that create PGE-2. Thus, PGE-3 is, by definition, an anti-inflammatory. Omega-3 fatty acids also increase detoxification enzyme activity (or Phase 2 enzymes) in animals. Detoxification enzymes are the body's built-in defense mechanism: they break down a variety of toxins, from pesticides to hormones. For instance, fish oil has been shown to protect against acetaminophen-induced (as found in Tylenol) liver injury by increasing the detoxification of the drug through Phase 2 enzymes.

In this discussion of omega-3 fatty acids and fish oils, we haven't yet menioned the one form of omega-3 that isn't fishy at all. It's called alpha-linolenic acid, and its main representatives are certain

---

The Other Fats and Cancer

It used to be commonplace to tell people that saturated fats caused cancer. Unfortunately, much of the research of the 1990s has shown that polyunsaturated fats, the kind you find in most vegetable oils, can also encourage it. The most commonly consumed vegetable oils, such as corn and sunflower oils, contain high levels of polyunsaturated omega-6 fatty acids. Omega-6 fatty acids, as opposed to omega-3 fatty acids, appear to promote colon cancer in laboratory animals. Therefore, I encourage people to be moderate in the use of both saturated and polyunsaturated fats. It is much safer, for instance, to cook with olive oil and avoid both butter and corn oil.

It is also clearly advisable to lower your consumption of red meats. Their relation to certain cancers—especially colon and prostate cancers—seems quite clear and is partially due to their high content of omega-6 fatty acids. Chicken and fish make far better animal-food entrées.

Pharmacist's Corner

■ If you dislike eating fish, try using flaxseed oil on your salad. The dosage would be about 1 ounce or 2 tablespoons daily.

■ Flaxseed oil turns rancid easily, so keep it in your refrigerator. You can tell if it goes rancid because its typically mild flavor will become much stronger. Because flaxseed oil turns rancid easily, you cannot cook with it.

■ The oils in high-potency fish-oil capsules are sometimes obtained by washing the oil with the toxic alcohol methanol. Solgar Vitamins offers a very high quality concentrated fish-oil supplement, Omega-3 700, which has a very high content of eicosapentaenoic acid (EPA) and docosahexaenoic acid (DHA) that has not been washed with methanol. Fish oils are also available in capsules under the trademark Maxepa and the minimum dosage is 1,000 milligrams 3 times daily with food.

■ Fish oil capsules can cause indigestion in some people. If this happens to you, switch to flaxseed oil or try using DHA from plankton 100 milligrams 3 times daily with food.

vegetable oils that aren't used much in the United States, including flaxseed, hempseed, cattail seed, and various other oils from nuts. Used for dietary supplementation, these oils, particularly flaxseed (also known as linseed) oil, can be wonderful additions to your diet. (Don't use these oils for cooking; store them in a dark jar or container under refrigeration.) Another benefit of these oils, some studies seem to suggest, is that alpha-linolenic acid provides particular protection against breast cancer.

Whether you supplement with flaxseed or increase your fish consumption, you will be doing yourself a favor—and not only in terms of cancer protection. Much research has demonstrated that omega-3 fatty acids lower blood pressure. Epidemiologic studies have shown that diets high in fish oil also decrease the risk of cardiovascular disease. This is partially because omega-3 fatty acids lower two kinds of fat that contribute to heart disease: triglycerides and very low density lipoprotein (VLDL) cholesterol.

I imagine the thrust of this chapter is pretty clear: eat more fish. The fish you should concentrate on eating most is the high-fat, omega-3 fish from the cold northern waters of the world: tuna, salmon, mackerel, cod, sardine, eel, halibut, and herring. Not only will they provide the benefits I've outlined above but they'll also provide you with copious quantities of vitamin D, a nutrient that researchers have found helps ward off breast cancer in postmenopausal women, as well as vitamin A, the immune-factor vitamin.

If you can acquire a real taste for seafood, you might find yourself eating 5 to 10 helpings of the marine critters weekly. It would be a great idea and a very useful part of any cancer prevention plan. High fish consumption is one of several critical factors that many epidemiologists believe explain the remarkably low rates of cancer in Japan.

CHAPTER
8

SOY AND GENISTEIN

*We have firmer ground to stand upon with
soy foods than any chemical.*

—STEVEN CLINTON, M.D., PH.D.,
Researcher at The
Dana Farber Cancer Institute in Boston

In the United States, the home of massive soybean crops and the world's major exporter of the food, soy remains an outcast at the dinner table. Soy burgers are not high on the list of delicacies at the average outdoor barbecue, and as far as most Americans are concerned, tofu is no food.

It doesn't need to be that way: soy can be quite tasty. Here and now, I will make the following prediction: simple self-preservation will eventually prompt us to pursue an up-front and personal relationship with the humble soybean. That's because soybeans, bless them, are packed with substances that we can pretty clearly identify as among the premier cancer killers in the human diet.

There are so many ways in which the natural chemicals in soy fight cancer . . . but, no, let me introduce you to a few statistics first. America's breast cancer rate is 22.4 per 100,000 people, which is nearly four times Japan's rate of 6 per 100,000. America's prostate cancer rate is 15.7 per 100,000 people, yet again four times Japan's rate of 3.5 per 100,000. Now, remaining aware that mere coincidence of numbers does not prove anything, let us look at soy consumption. The Japanese consume 30 to 50 times more soy products than do Americans. When the urinary excretion of certain phytoestrogens found in soy—primarily genistein and diadzen—were measured in Japanese women and American women, the Japanese women excreted 2,000 to 3,000 nanomolar per day, and the American women, 30 to 40 nanomolar per day. Translation: the soybean abyss is probably the most dramatic difference between the Japanese and the American diets.

Now let's look at the reasons why more and more scientists think soy is behind much of that fourfold difference between the breast and prostate cancer rates of the two countries.

Soy, one of the richest sources of protein in the plant kingdom, contains biologically active compounds called isoflavones that have been shown to have a startlingly wide range of activity in the body. These substances—genistein, diadzen, and glycitein, three of the most common varieties—are phytoestrogens; that is, they are plant estrogens. Extensive research has demonstrated that the isoflavones found in soy can lower cholesterol levels, regulate hormonal balance in women, stop hot flashes, keep the tissues of the vagina healthy and moist after menopause, help prevent osteoporosis, and protect against cancer by a startling variety of different modes of operation. We may eventually conclude that the isoflavones—genistein in particular—are nature's own anticancer medication, and we won't even have had to go into the Amazon jungle to find it. Let's look at the range of effects that soy and its finest isoflavone, genistein, have at their command.

STARVING THE CANCER

Cancers don't grow without blood. They need their very own supply, and they reach out to get it. They tap into a natural process of the body—angiogenesis, which is the creation of new blood vessels. Actually, once you've gotten into adulthood, your body doesn't have much need for this process unless you're pregnant or healing from some injury. Nonetheless, the process is there, and for a tumor, the need is no different. The stage at which a system of new blood vessels begins to grow around it, so that it can be supplied with all the nutrients it needs to grow and prosper at your expense, is a crucial one. Until sufficient cells in the cancer mass learn how to promote the creation of new blood vessels, the malignancy will remain small and vulnerable.

Cancer researchers have long hoped to find a way to halt the process of angiogenesis in tumors. The spasm of excitement over shark cartilage several years ago was based on the idea that it would do just that, but, to date, medical research has not found any basis for those hopes.

Science has shown, however, that diets rich in soy have been associated with the prevention of new blood vessel growth. A 1993 European study, for example, found potent antiangiogenesis blockers containing high concentrations of genistein in the urine of people eating a diet rich in soy. A German study and a recent study from Johns Hopkins University in Baltimore have also shown that genistein prevents the growth of blood vessel cells in lab cultures. These findings make it seem very likely that we have an angiogenesis inhibitor available in our grocery stores.

DISARMING THE CANCER

In the total economy of the human body, cancer cells are evil geniuses capable of fooling, fouling, and flummoxing the security forces of your metabolism. One of their tricks is to produce high levels of stress proteins to defend themselves from the attacks that your immune system will launch against them once it identifies their abnormality. These proteins are called glucose-related proteins (GRPs) and heat shock proteins (HSPs), the latter of which buffer cancer cells against stressful, high-temperature conditions.

It turns out that genistein has the happy attribute of suppressing the production of stress proteins. This is bad news for a cancer. Robbed of its chemical shield, a small cancer stands a very good chance of succumbing to your immune system long before you or your doctor even knows about it.

In a 1998 study published in the *Journal of the National Cancer Institute,* the author noted not only that "the anti-cancer effects of genistein may be related to its abilities to reduce the expression of stress response–related genes" but also that by this mechanism, genistein might formidably enhance the anticancer effects of chemotherapy and radiation. Stress protein production is central to the system whereby a robust cancer survives exactly such stressful assaults on its vital integrity.

Since medicine is always looking for treatments that work synergistically with time-tested therapies of one sort or another, I'm expecting to see soybean research increase sharply as a result of that report.

ZAPPING THE CANCER

Yet another enzyme in the body, protein-tyrosine kinase, has been shown to be necessary for a tumor to grow. Tyrosine kinase helps prevent natural cell death. When a cell grows old or mutates, a process of programmed cell death occurs; the process is called apoptosis. In order to remain juvenile delinquents forever, cancer cells must work around apoptosis. Tyrosine kinase is an important cell-signaling molecule that when activated, helps confer immortality on cancer cells.

Researchers have found, however, that isoflavones—particularly genistein—block the activation of tyrosine kinase. In 1996, researchers demonstrated that in this manner, genistein was capable of inhibiting prostate cancer cell growth.

TAKING AWAY CANCER'S FRIENDS

Now we'll discuss a mechanism of activity in soy and its special isoflavone, genistein, that explains its remarkable effectiveness at preventing breast cancer and possibly other cancers as well. Soy is a type of plant food that is referred to as a phytoestrogen—that is, a plant estrogen. This simply means that chemically its components, such as genistein and diadzen, are very similar to the female sex hormone estrogen. When compared with the very potent estrogen, however, these isoflavone plant estrogens seem to be weaker and to have little estrogenic activity. In fact, researchers have concluded that they are only $\frac{1}{1,000}$ as powerful as estrogen.

As you're probably aware, high levels of estrogen are believed to increase breast cancer risk. Indeed, they may also increase the risk of prostate, uterine, and colon cancers, since the prostate, uterus, and colon have shown to have fairly numerous estrogen receptors. Receptor sites on cells are sort of like docks specially fitted to receive particular molecular ships when they arrive in port. If there are no receptor sites for estrogen or if the sites are occupied by something else, then estrogen simply won't make a landfall on that particular cell.

The great significance of this is that the weakly estrogenic isoflavones found in soy are similar enough to estrogen to be welcome at its cellular receptor sites. If enough soy isoflavones are circulating in the body, they will tend to hog the available receptors, thus effectively blocking estrogen. As a result, the more years a woman spends on a high-soy diet, the lower her lifetime cellular exposure to the much more potent estrogen of her own body.

Help for Men, Too

Men have become unhappily aware of their prostate gland since the early 1990s. This little chesnut-size organ that produces the liquid portion of semen is all too frequently big trouble as we age. It often causes urinary problems due to a condition known as benign prostatic hypertrophy (BPH), and it also causes cancer on a large scale. With prostate cancer's death rate being higher than 40,000 men a year, only lung cancer takes a bigger slice from the male half of the population.

Prostate cancer is unusual in that frequently, enclosed within the capsule of the prostate gland, the tumor can exist for years or decades without spreading or otherwise endangering the man who has it. A recent comparison of autopsy studies done on Asian and Western men who died of other causes revealed that the incidence of such hidden prostate cancer was virtually the same in the two groups, yet it has been known for decades that the incidence of fatal prostate cancer is far higher among Western men than Asian men. The reasons are almost certainly related to diet: (1) vegetable consumption, (2) fat consumption, and (3) soy consumption.

Not only does soy have the variety of anticancer activities that we've pointed out, but men also benefit from its estrogen-controlling proclivities in surprising ways. Estrogen is believed to stimulate cell growth in the prostate gland, just as it does in women's breasts. Many men don't realize that they have significant levels of estrogen in their bloodstream, just as women have significant levels of the male hormone, testosterone. Interestingly, men get their estrogen mostly from testosterone. There is an enzyme in the human body called aromatase that converts testosterone to estrogen. The main phytoestrogen in soy—genistein—happens to be a particularly effective inhibitor of aromatase. In other words, with enough phytoestrogens at your command, your body will not only block estrogen receptor sites but also prevent estrogen's manufacture in the first place.

Soy's effects on women's reproductive hormone levels is so marked that the length of a woman's menstrual cycle is altered on soy-rich diets. When women are given soy-based phytoestrogens, the length of their cycle increases by an average of 2.5 days, and such a longer menstrual cycle is associated with decreased risk of breast cancer.

It is also a fact—the basic fact relating estrogen to cancer risk—that estrogen promotes cell growth. A 1997 study of cell cultures emphatically demonstrated that genistein was unique among isoflavones not only in opposing estrogen at the cell receptor sites but in also strongly inhibiting cell growth. The particular cells the scientists were growing were breast cancer cells.

Genistein is probably the most powerfully effective phytoestrogen yet discovered. In addition to its abundance in soy, it is also found in high amounts in black beans, which may account for the reduced rates of breast cancer among Hispanic women.

STANDING IN THE STORM

Protection from breast cancer is the foremost benefit promised and delivered by our friend the soybean. American women are all too well aware that they stand in the midst of a veritable epidemic of breast cancer. There are many reasons for this, including the longest period between puberty and menopause ever seen in human history, low rates of childbearing, environmental exposures to chemical estrogens (xenoestrogens), and simple longevity. Scientists and polemicists will argue about which cause to emphasize, but the end result is, alas, all too clear: today, one American woman in nine gets breast cancer at some time in her life.

In fact, more than 200,000 women get breast cancer yearly. Almost 50,000 die of it. Survival rates for women in whom the cancer has metastasized have not significantly improved since the 1960s, either. To be the owner of breasts in America today is to stand in the midst of the whirlwind.

There is another interesting fact about breast cancer: it is one of the cancers whose incidence changes dramatically when people migrate and alter dietary habits, abandoning old food traditions and taking up new ones. When Asian women move from China or Japan and come to America, for example, they acquire the vastly higher American level of breast cancer risk in less than a generation. It is believed that a higher level of fat in their new diet is part of the problem, but that is probably not the whole story. As you're about to see, declining level of soy consumption is very likely to be another highly significant piece of the puzzle (as is a decline in the consumption of green tea and the cold-water fish that are rich in omega-3 fatty acids).

Here is some of the research that justifies calling soy your friend:

- A study found that Seventh Day Adventist women, vegetarians with high soy intake, had a lower risk of breast cancer combined with higher levels of DHEA (dihydroepiandrosterone), an adrenal androgen that has been found before to be present in generally higher levels in women who are free of breast cancer.
- An Italian study at the University of Milan found that the combination of genistein and an anticancer drug called Adriamycin showed an increased, syngeristic effectiveness in halting human breast cancer cell proliferation.
- In a 1989 study of 8,000 Hawaiian men of Japanese ancestry, those who ate the most tofu had the lowest rates of prostate cancer. A Shanghai study found that women who seldom ate soy foods had twice the rate of breast cancer of those who ate soy frequently.

Animal research supports these powerful indications of soy's benefits:

- A 1995 study on rats found that cell proliferation leading to mammary cancer (the rodent equivalent of breast cancer) was sharply reduced in genistein-treated rats. The results were particularly striking when the soy isoflavone was given to rats before puberty. It was found that genistein occupied estrogen receptor sites. The authors concluded that "genistein exerts its action via the estrogen receptor mechanism, that in turn sets in motion a cascade of downstream events to result in gland differentiation and less susceptibility for mammary cancer."
- Lab studies with animals show that soy milk inhibits the formation of mammary tumors. In one study, already established tumors in female rats showed significantly slower growth when the rats were switched from cow's milk to soy milk as their main source of protein.
- Scientists compared the blood levels of soy isoflavonoids in Japanese men with those of Finnish men, who have higher

rates of prostate cancer. The Japanese men's blood contained from 7 to 110 times as much isoflavonoids, suggesting that the higher levels protect men from prostate cancer.

GO FOR THE SOY

Are all the studies described in this chapter sufficient evidence of the unique merits of the soybean? I hope so. Soy deserves a book; I'm embarrassed to give it only a chapter.

My suggestion is that you begin using soy milk, tofu, miso (a form of soy paste), and tempeh, a fermented soy patty that has a nutty, "mushroomy," meatlike flavor and texture that makes it perfect for marinating, grilling, searing, or baking. Find a good cookbook with a large section on soy. It's actually not difficult to get used to the taste, and most people who eat soy for a while find that they like it.

You, too, can become a consumer of the most widely eaten plant in the world. Then you could find yourself acquiring, along with the culinary habits of the Asians, their lower cancer rates.

Soy Sources

Soy milk:
- Extracted from dried soybeans
- Comes in a variety of flavors, from chocolate to strawberry
- Can be found in most supermarkets and health-food stores

Tofu:
- Made from the curd of soy milk
- Is cholesterol free and protein rich
- Can be used in soups and salads or as a substitute for meat, as in tofu burgers

Soy yogurt:
- Is yogurt made with bacterial cultures and soy milk
- Is an excellent low-fat substitute for dairy yogurt
- Can be found in most health-food stores

Miso:
- Is flavored soy paste fermented with rice and salt
- Makes wonderful soups and salad dressings

Soy protein extracts:
- Are an excellent source of all soy isflavones
- Are found in designer foods and energy bars
- May be used in juicing, milk shakes, or baking

Soy food substitutes:
- Come in the forms of protein- and isoflavone-rich soy-based hamburgers, sausages, and cheeses (with flavors from mozzarella to cheddar)
- Are excellent low-fat alternatives to beef and dairy products

Soy flour:
- Is made from ground roasted soybeans
- Is an excellent source of isoflavones and protein
- Is great for adding to bread flour or baked goods

Soy sauce:
- Is made from fermenting soybeans with wheat and mold
- Is a soy form from which, unfortunately, all isoflavones are processed out
- Is very tasty but has a high salt content
- Intake does not give you the benefits of soy

Soybean oils:
- Are a soy form from which all isoflavones are lost in processing
- Are rich in linolenic acids, which can be converted to omega-3 fatty acids
- Are a second choice when you run out of olive oil or need an oil without flavor

Pharmacist's Corner

■ It is estimated that we need to eat about 8 ounces of soy foods daily. This may be impractical for many of us. You can supplement your intake of soy foods by taking a 500- to 1,000-milligram soy isoflavonoid supplement once or even twice daily that contains 12 to 20 milligrams of genestein and diadzein per dose.

■ Soy foods and rice contain phytates. Vegetarians who consume large amounts of soy and rice should consider mineral supplementation because phytates can attach to the zinc, copper, and calcium in other foods and prevent their absorption. If you are on this type of diet you might want to see a licensed nutritionist for advice on mineral replacement. This is not a problem with extracted soy isoflavonoid supplements.

■ **Possible drug interaction:** Soybeans contain some vitamin K. Vitamin K can interfere somewhat with the lifesaving effects of the anticoagulant drug warfarin (Coumadin). If you are taking this drug and want to add soy foods to your diet, you must inform your doctor.

■ For information on soy foods, a list of the ingredients, guidance on which soy supplements to take, or a list of the advantages and disadvantages of taking soy protein, visit us at our web site at **www.jerryhickey.com** or contact us at our e-mail address: **hickeychemists@jerryhickey.com**.

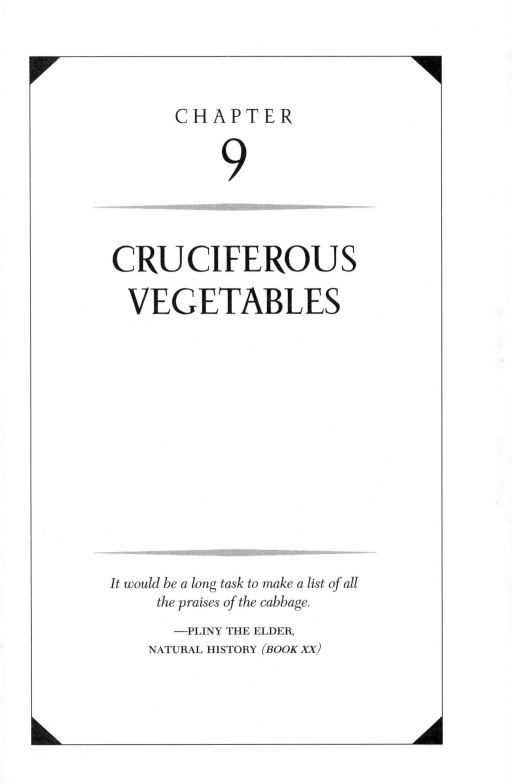

CHAPTER

9

CRUCIFEROUS VEGETABLES

It would be a long task to make a list of all the praises of the cabbage.

—PLINY THE ELDER,
NATURAL HISTORY *(BOOK XX)*

Go ahead, spear one of those pungent brussels sprouts. Dip into the cabbage soup. Crunch down on a broccoli tree. I don't know whether I've aroused or depressed your appetite, but I'm sure of one thing: the instinct of self-preservation, which by repute is active in almost everyone, will lead you to dig into cruciferous veggies yet.

These little fellas are big provokers of anticancer enzymes, and there are medical studies to prove it. Doctors and scientists under the direction of Leon Bradlow, Ph.D., at Strang Cancer Prevention Center found that many children with recurrent vocal cord polyps have had complete resolution of this condition when given a regular regimen of cabbage juice. As early as ancient Rome, people were already aware that cabbage seemed to make people healthy, and Pliny the Elder noted that among its uses was as a treatment for cancerous sores "which can be healed by no other treatment." It—like bok choy, broccoli, brussels sprouts, kale, and cauliflower—is called a cruciferous vegetable. *Cruciferous* comes from the word for crucifying or placing on a cross; cruciferous plants' flowers contain two components that can be arranged like a cross.

What all such veggies have in common from a phytonutrient standpoint are certain natural chemicals that have extremely discouraging effects on cancer cells. These are sulfur-containing compounds, the thiocyanates; some of the better-known substances that have been isolated from them include the indoles and sulforaphane. Sulfur, as you may remember from high-school chemistry, has a distinctive odor, and cooking the cruciferous vegetables produces a smell that some people find unpleasant. President George Bush, as you might recall, was clearly in a quandary about whether it was broccoli or Saddam Hussein he disliked most of all.

For the purpose of this book, though, I'm not going to say

anything but good things about cruciferous vegetables from now on. Numerous studies have found with astonishing consistency that people who eat them lower their risk of cancer. This really isn't news anymore. A case-control study of colon cancer in Japan way back in 1980 found that people who ate high amounts of the cruciferous team radically lowered their risk for the malignancy.

In 1996, Dutch scientists summarized the research from 94 clinical trials and large population studies that have addressed the question of cruciferous consumption and cancer risk. Sixty-seven percent of the studies showed that consumption of any of the cruciferous vegetables decreased the rate of cancers at various sites. In the total scheme of things, cabbage, broccoli, and cauliflower showed the highest protective effects, with brussels sprouts' effects being somewhat lower. The Dutch analysis showed that the most consistent protective effects were racked up against lung, stomach, colon, and rectal cancers. Rates for prostatic, endometrial, and ovarian cancers were not significantly affected.

Looking for the truth in this matter, other researchers turned their attention to rats and mice. In 1994, the folks at Johns Hopkins University in Baltimore decided to infuse sulforaphane into rats. This team, headed by Paul Talalay, Ph.D., and Gary Posner, Ph.D., had isolated the chemical from broccoli two years earlier and showed by experimentation in laboratory dishes that it stimulated the growth of anticancer enzymes. Then they injected 29 rats with either a low or a high dose of sulforaphane. Afterward, they gave the rats a shot of dimethylbenzantracene (DMBA), a carcinogen that causes mammary tumors (the rat equivalent of breast cancer). Another 25 rats, chosen to be experimental controls, were simply given the carcinogen without the sulforaphane.

The two groups of rodents fared very differently. In the group on DMBA alone, 68 percent came down with breast cancer. Those receiving sulforaphane at the lower dose had a 35 percent cancer incidence and, of those on a high dose, only 26 percent contracted cancer. Even those among the sulforaphane rats that did get cancer did so later than members of the untreated group, and their tumors were smaller and fewer in number.

STIMULATE YOUR BODY'S OWN DEFENSES

Cleaning out your toxic garbage is the special activity of the Phase 2 detoxification enzymes that I introduced you to in Chapter 4. It appears that sulforaphane's major anticancer function is to stimulate those enzymes. It's a particularly vigorous member of a group of stimulators called the isothiocyanates, as demonstrated in studies of rat and mouse tissues. In fact, sulforaphane has induced production of two powerful Phase 2 enzymes, quinone reductase and glutathione transferase, in rat and mouse tissues. Compounds like sulforaphane probably don't have much in the way of nutritional value. It's their power of enzymatic stimulation that has value for human health. Recently, scientists at Johns Hopkins have been developing synthetic analogues of sulforaphane that may be equally effective. We await results here with some eagerness.

INDOLES AGAINST BREAST CANCER

Meanwhile, a whole host of animal and cell culture studies are showing that some of the indoles in the cruciferous vegetables—particularly indole-3-carbinol (I3C)—are potent antagonists of breast cancer.

Researchers in Texas, for example, found that I3C could block a receptor site in breast cancer cells, causing a 90 percent reduction in stimulating further cancerous activity. It was assumed here that the basis of this reduction was I3C's ability to occupy sites that would otherwise be occupied by estrogen.

Further investigations have confirmed this. Using a culture of breast cancer cells, one team of researchers specifically examined I3C's effect on estrogen-responsive cells. You see, not all the cells in a woman's breast are responsive to estrogen or have estrogen receptor sites where the female hormone can land, but the ones that are so responsive are particularly important to the development of breast cancer. It was found that I3C specifically inhibited the development of estrogen-responsive cells. This selectivity may explain the ability of cruciferous vegetables to lower the risk of breast cancer.

This doesn't appear to be the only way, however, that I3C can reduce a woman's risk from estrogen. Estrogen is actually a number of different hormones, estradiol, estrone, and estriol being the most important forms. In the early 1990s, researchers discovered that I3C was capable of altering the metabolism of estradiol, the most potent and carcinogenic form of estrogen. It's almost entirely estradiol that doctors worry about when they see high concentrations of it in human breast tissue. Lower levels of dietary fat, aerobic exercise, weight loss, and, ironically, cigarette smoking have also all been shown to decrease estradiol levels.

The I3C from cruciferous vegetables is also an estradiol reducer, which is great news. In medical terms, there is a process called 2-hydroxylation that converts estradiol to estrone, a more benign form of the hormone. More estrone and less estradiol results in a reduced incidence of breast and endometrial cancer in women. The significance of this conversion is immensely enhanced by the fact that I3C is the only nutrient yet identified capable of converting estrogen from a cancer-enhancing to a cancer-preventing form. We appear to be dealing with a very powerful and almost unique process.

If more protection is necessary, I3C provides more. The levels of an important liver enzyme called cytochrome P450 increase after administration of the indole. Cytochrome P450 has the capacity to process estradiol and then excrete it.

As you've seen, the result of all this activity is to effectively lower levels of estradiol, the most carcinogenic form of estrogen.

Using I3C, researchers at both Strang Cancer Prevention Center and Rockefeller University in New York have shown experimentally that mammary tumor incidence became significantly lower in female mice whose chow contained the phytonutrient. They were also able to show increases in cytochrome P450 levels and increases in estradiol 2-hydroxylation. This evidence seems to impressively support the theoretical explanation for the effects of the cruciferous vegetables on breast cancer.

CRUCIFEROUS SPROUTS ARE COMING AT YOU

What if you simply can't stand the taste of cruciferous vegetables or you can't handle them more than once a week? Well, there may be an answer.

Pharmacist's Corner

■ If you do not like the taste of broccoli, try taking a 500-milligram capsule of broccoli supplement once or twice a day with meals. This supplement should have a guaranteed sulforaphane content equal to two 200-gram servings of broccoli or approximately 200 micrograms of sulforaphane. Broccoli also contains some carotenoids, indoles, and glutathione, all very healthy ingredients.

■ **Drug interaction:** Vegetables in the cabbage family contain vitamin K and they will interfere with the anticoagulant drug warfarin (Coumadin). If you are already eating these vegetables and your condition has stabilized with Coumadin, don't worry—your doctor is monitoring your prothrombin (blood clotting) time. If you are taking Coumadin and want to add these vegetables to your diet or increase the amount you are already consuming, however, you must work closely with your doctor. In some cases, your physician may believe it is impossible to add more vitamin K–containing vegetables to your diet. The vitamin K in these vegetables shortens your prothrombin time and can make the lifesaving drug Coumadin less effective.

■ Indole-3-carbinol (soon available in capsule form) is a good supplement to your diet of cruciferous vegetables. The dosage is 200 milligrams to 1,000 milligrams daily.

Scientists hunting for a way to increase the levels of sulforaphane and the Phase 2 enzyme detoxification activity it stimulates have turned their attention to 3-day-old broccoli sprouts. The sprouts are quite bland and don't taste like broccoli at all, but they contain from 20 to 50 times as much of a precursor of sulforaphane as mature broccoli does. Plans are under way to market the sprouts as an important health food.

Until we're lucky enough to be offered salvation by sprout, I'd suggest that you might want to try acquiring a taste for the crucifers. If you're fortunate enough to already like them, well then, dig in. Half a dozen servings of cruciferous vegetables weekly can only be good for you. Eating them raw in salads would be healthiest, but if you cook them, as most people do, steamed is best.

Another approach for those of you who don't love this branch of the plant kingdom is juicing. Take a third of a head of broccoli or a fourth of a head of cabbage and run it through a blender with two carrots. The result, pleasantly sweetened by the carrots, is more than just palatable. Who knows? You may become an enthusiast.

CHAPTER

10

HERBS AND BEES

Foolish is the doctor who despises the knowledge acquired by the ancients.

—HIPPOCRATES

F ar up the Congo River, somewhere in the depths of the jungle, perhaps on a steep, green hillside where the monkeys chatter, the birds chirp, and the leopards roar at night, there grows a herb that will certainly save you. Right? Well, maybe.

On the other hand, you might be looking in the wrong place. There are herbal miracles much closer to home and already discovered. You may not have to go to central Africa and search for an exotic plant or for the wingtip claw mold of the two-striped jungle bat. After all, nature's answers to our health problems are spread all around—just the way nature is. I'm not surprised that the herbs and spices that go into both American and Eastern cuisine are loaded with cancer fighters. These recipe stimulators don't just make dull foods taste good; they make lively people live longer.

This is an old story in medicine. Many traditional pharmaceuticals come from plants. Morphine and codeine come from poppy seeds; digitalis, a heart tonic, comes from the foxglove flower; taxol, an important chemotherapeutic agent, comes from the yew tree; and quinine, the original antimalarial drug, comes from the bark of the cinchona tree. In 1990, it was estimated that there were 121 prescription drugs derived from plants.

In addition, of course, folk medicine is full of herbal remedies, and doctors who come to medicine with a conservative, traditional training—and we almost all have—can easily be surprised at the effectiveness of those approaches. You know most of these herbs by name. They're in every cookbook and, in all probability, they represent at least several of these very common substances that you drop into your stew pot or your casserole now and then. Healthy herbs—herbs that have anticarcinogenic effects—are a common part of the human diet in most cultures, including ours.

This chapter is a potpourri of remarkable and often very flavor-

111

ful herbal friends. Try adding a few of these phytonutrient flavor enhancers to your personal cuisine. They could turn out to be strong medicine. In this chapter's last section, we will make a little detour into the realm of the bee. This common insect appears to be the keeper of some of nature's secrets.

ROSEMARY

Rosemary is a spice whose anticarcinogenic properties are rapidly becoming evident. I invariably give rosemary to patients who come to me for cancer prevention. It is nontoxic, has valuable antioxidant properties, and, as you will shortly see, has provoked a series of intriguing scientific studies.

This common spice comes from the plant *rosmarinus officinalis,* native to the Mediterranean. Certainly, it has been used as a flavoring agent since ancient times. Apart from its other valuable properties, it also has fair to good concentrations of calcium, magnesium, and potassium.

In studies done in the 1990s, researchers have found that rosemary is a powerful inhibitor of tumors, a promoter of detoxification enzymes, and a potent inhibitor of the cyclooxygenase-2 (COX-2) enzyme, that dangerous ally of undesirable prostaglandins that I talked about in Chapter 3 when I explained the immune system.

This herb's most important quality is the ability to produce a major increase in the activity of two helpful enzymes: glutathione-S-transferase and quinone reductase. You might want to look back for a moment to Chapter 4, where we discussed these magnificent natural protectors. In our very dirty world, a good detoxification enzyme is a friend indeed. Scientists at the University of Illinois demonstrated this in rats by raising rats' levels of glutathione-S-transferase six times above the normal when given an extract of rosemary. For its part, quinone reductase was simultaneously increased two- to fourfold.

Stimulation of such enzymes certainly ought to offer some protection against cancer. In fact, the rats have shown it's so. In one study out of Rutgers University in New Jersey, skin tumors were reduced by 54 percent to 64 percent by the use of a rosemary ex-

Pharmacist's Corner

■ Rosemary is available as a tea or leaf extract. For any herbal tea, steep the tea bag in hot water for 3 minutes, then squeeze the juice left in the bag into the cup. Try brewing a mixture of rosemary, orange, and green teas together and drink a cup three times a day.

■ Rosemary leaf extract is in a weak alcohol base; use 10 drops three times daily in tea.

tract. Another study by the same team of scientists reduced breast and colon tumors by 45 percent and 85 percent, respectively, using this savory herb.

Rosemary does more than promote detoxification. Several studies have shown that there are compounds in rosemary that can block carcinogenic chemicals from binding to deoxyribonucleic acid (DNA) in cells. This means that this spicy little number can call a halt to unwelcome changes right at the gates of carcinogenic catastrophe. That ability may be why a study conducted on human bronchial cancer cells demonstrated that the herb could block the cancer production that would normally be caused by benzoprene, one of the chief chemicals in cigarette smoke. It could be that that bowl of curry that I recommended for smokers (see page 123) will eventually be flavored with rosemary.

Rosemary has not yet been tested in studies of human populations to see if its use is associated with long-term cancer prevention, and it is not known what levels will provide protection. Nonetheless, I think you should introduce rosemary into your diet and keep your eye out for further reports. This is going to be a well-researched plant product in years to come.

GINSENG

Ginseng, the famous star of Oriental herbalism, has a role in cancer prevention. If reports from South Korea are confirmed by other researchers, that role may be enormous.

There are a variety of different herbs that are marketed under the name *ginseng* with greater or lesser authenticity. The true source of the major representative of the ginseng family is the plant *Panax ginseng,* often called Chinese ginseng. *Panax ginseng* is currently grown in Korea, Japan, and China. This small perennial woodlands plant has been used in Oriental medicine for more than 5,000 years and has been most thoroughly researched. The effects of American ginseng (*Radix panacis quinquefolii*) are not nearly so well established, and Siberian ginseng is in fact derived not from ginseng at all but rather from an edible plant known as *Eleuthrococcus senticosus,* so we won't discuss them here.

There are a number of compounds in ginseng, the most important of which appear to be the dozen or so ginseng saponins. Traditionally, people have used ginseng to increase strength, vitality, and appetite and to help in dealing with stress. An interesting concept has been applied to ginseng, the idea that it is an "adaptogen." This means a substance that helps the body adapt to age or disease by doing whatever is necessary to maintain the proper balancing of all systems. A scientist would call such a state of healthy equilibrium homeostasis; if indeed ginseng promotes it, that might help to explain its health-enhancing effects. It also has potent antioxidant capacities that may help.

Meanwhile, of all the studies done on ginseng and cancer, only a series conducted in Seoul, Korea, by T. K. Yun, Ph.D., directly deals with its effects on humans. This research is an eye opener. For five years, Dr. Yun monitored 4,634 people in areas of Korea where ginseng is produced. Ginseng consumers had approximately 50 percent the likelihood of contracting cancer that nonconsumers had. The probability was dose- and duration-related, meaning the more ginseng people consumed and the longer they had been taking it, the more their cancer risk fell. Also, ginseng extract was found to provide more potent protection than did slices of ginseng or ginseng tea.

Dr. Yun did a further study on 1,987 people in 1995. This was what is called a case-control study: a patient without cancer is studied for each patient with cancer and a comparison of various factors is made. The results for ginseng were very similar to those of the earlier study. Patients who had been taking ginseng for one year had a 36 percent lower cancer incidence than did nonconsumers of the herb; patients who had been taking it for five years or more had 69 percent less. Ginseng showed the most protective effect against cancer of the ovaries, larynx, esophagus, pancreas, and stomach. There seemed to be no significant effect on breast, bladder, thyroid, and cervical cancers.

These fairly sizable human studies have been backed up by animal research. In one case, in which liver cancer was induced in rats by a carcinogen, only 14 percent of the rats given ginseng extract got the cancer, while 100 percent of the unprotected rats did. In another study, the rate of lung tumors induced in mice decreased after the administration of ginseng and the level of natural killer cells went up.

One final note: researchers at Harvard have shown that ginseng is a phytoestrogen and may occupy estrogen receptor sites. In the process, it may cause certain favorable estrogenic changes in the body that have been associated with decreased breast cancer risk. Indeed, along the lines already observed in soy foods, ginseng may prove to be an important antagonist to breast cancer.

Pharmacist's Corner

■ *Panax ginseng* is readily available from many dependable manufacturers. Bulk materials of Panax ginseng, however, have been removed from distribution because of pesticide contamination. Mariposa, a quality herbal manufacturer, is a good source for pesticide and fungus-free Panax ginseng. Take one 100 milligram capsule of guaranteed-potency Korean *Panax ginseng* once or twice a day with food. Some herbal practitioners advise patients to follow a rotating schedule of 3 weeks on and 1 week off of *Panax ginseng;* however, there don't seem to be any studies supporting this break in the schedule.

■ In rare instances, *Panax ginseng* can cause overstimulation, and this effect can be exacerbated by coffee.

LICORICE

Licorice is considered to be the most important constituent in Chinese traditional medicine after ginseng and is used in even more formulations. The herb is grown widely throughout China, Russia, southern Europe, and the Middle East. The Japanese absorb a sizable part of the world's production, importing more than 9,000 tons a year.

Licorice has a wide variety of activities, many of them based on its capacity to diminish inflammation in various parts of the body. It appears to soothe stomach upset, discourage allergic reactions, and provide some relief for arthritis. In the 1960s, an article in the *Journal of Pharmacy and Pharmacology* demonstrated that the herb possessed a cough-suppressing ability equal to that of codeine, a mild narcotic.

These anti-inflammatory properties probably play a role in the herb's apparent cancer prevention effects. The inflammation-causing compounds that licorice inhibits are also suspects in the causation of certain kinds of cancer. The herb that we call licorice is the sweet-tasting root of the plant glycyrrhiza (*Radix glycyrrhiza uralensis*). That sweet taste is produced by compounds called triterpenoids. Most research on licorice has used licorice-root extracts. In the most impressive study so far conducted, licorice

Pharmacist's Corner

■ Licorice is available in tea bags, capsules, and drops. The problem with licorice is that its antitumor ingredients resemble a class of hormones known as mineralocorticoids, which have the effect of increasing blood pressure, causing a loss of potassium, with a corresponding retention of sodium and water, resulting in swelling. Because licorice in relatively modest doses will cause these symptoms and because it's not unusual for a person eating lots of licorice candy to experience these effects, have only 1 cup of licorice tea or less than 350 milligrams of the encapsulated herb daily.

proved highly effective in preventing tumors in mice. Scientists promoted lung and stomach tumors in a group of female mice, simultaneously giving one half of them a licorice extract to drink. The mice who had been dosed with licorice registered a 20 percent drop in lung tumor incidence and a 60 percent drop in total number of tumors (many of the affected mice had more than one tumor). There was also a 33 percent drop in stomach cancer incidence among the licorice-treated mice.

There is another chemical in licorice: licochalcone. After isolating the chemical, researchers applied it topically on mice in which they had initiated skin cancer. In the group not treated with licochalcone, 73.3 percent of the mice had tumors after 20 weeks. In the treated group, only 26.7 percent developed tumors over the course of the study. It is believed that licochalcone is a substance that can inhibit ultraviolet (UV) radiation-induced DNA changes.

One last study done at the University of Texas in 1997 demonstrated that licorice extract could lower the rate of metastases from the deadliest of skin cancers—melanomas—by 78 percent, once again in mice.

The evidence is very encouraging, and I have been urging patients for some time now to include licorice in their diet. Nonetheless, caution is advised here. See the Pharmacist's Corner (page 116) on licorice for more information on its correct use.

GINGER

Ginger, a delightful diet constituent in many parts of the world, is yet another spice that seems to possess cancer-preventive properties.

Fresh ginger is a brown, knobby root that originally came from southeast Asia and has a paperlike covering. It can be consumed fresh or used in powdered, pickled, or crystalized form. Oils extracted from ginger have been found to increase some of the detoxification enzymes that our bodies depend on. The herb also contains powerful antioxidants called gingerol and zingerone. Japanese scientists have identified 14 compounds in ginger that are stronger antioxidants than vitamin E. This undoubtedly explains

> ### ◤ *Pharmacist's* Corner
>
> ■ Among ginger's many properties is its usefulness in treating nausea and gastric distress, but in high doses, along the order of taking two 550-milligram capsules two to four times daily. We need far less ginger for its antioxidant effect; one 550-milligram capsule once or twice daily is plenty. Ginger tea is tasty; 2 to 3 cups daily offers a good supply of antioxidants.

why, prior to modern canning and refrigeration, ginger was often used in traditional cultures as a preservative: its antioxidant properties helped to protect food from oxidative stress and subsequent spoilage.

Those antioxidant properties would be reason enough for you to include ginger in your lifetime anticancer plan. A recent animal study encourages that view. Researchers in Cleveland gave ginger extract to mice in which they were promoting skin cancer. Guess what? There was a significant drop in tumor formation among the ginger-protected mice.

I think ginger will be better researched in the West in coming years. At the moment, I still have no hesitation in recommending it highly for its known properties—and remember it has been in use in the East for thousands of years.

SESAME

Sesame seed and sesame oil have been popular health foods for some time. They also have a long history of use in the cuisines of Africa, India, and China. Tahini, a spread sometimes called the "butter of the Middle East," is made from ground sesame seeds. It's now used as a delicious salad dressing in health-conscious restaurants and is found in the ever more popular food, hummus.

Why have sesame seed and sesame oil been regarded as healthy? Well, possibly because recent research shows that their antioxidant potential is formidable. Certain lignan compounds

Pharmacist's Corner

- Sesame is available in capsule form and helps supply antioxidants. Because of the number of foods and nutrients described in this book, however, it may be impractical to take each one separately. A solution can involve ingesting them in designer foods and medical foods that supply a broad combination of available nutrients. Oncologics provides such items.

unique to sesame, as well as tocopherol and other antioxidant substances, make this a very potent herb with obvious anticancer potential.

ECHINACEA

Echinacea is an herb that is native to North America, once flourishing in our prairies and woodlands. Native Americans and the colonists from Europe used this herb to counter a large variety of illnesses, particularly fevers and infections. To this day, herbalists prescribe extracts of echinacea to give a quick boost when the immune system is under siege.

It would appear that the secret of its effects are its large polysaccharides, such as inulin. These stimulate the production of mac-

Pharmacist's Corner

- Echinacea is usually taken in capsule form as an immune system enhancement. People with minor complaints, however, do better with an Enchinacea tincture. A typical dosage for capsules is one 350- to 550-milligram capsule four times daily for a 3-week cycle, with a 1-week break in between. The tincture is usually taken if you have the flu or a cold, at a dose of 30 drops three times a day in some orange juice.

rophages and, as German scientists have shown in a number of studies, two other immune system components—natural killer cells and neutrophils.

Naturally, this ability could have a positive effect in dealing with cancer. For example, a 1981 study demonstrated that the polysaccharides in echinacea significantly increased the killing effect of macrophages on tumor cells. In a study of patients with inoperable metastatic esophageal or colorectal cancer, natural killer cell activity increased, happily, by 221 percent after the use of echinacea. Traditionally, however, echinacea is not used for long periods without a break. I think we can say that this is a powerful substance but that the jury is still out on its usefulness as a cancer preventive agent. Research is badly needed here.

MILK THISTLE

Milk thistle, which contains a potent group of flavonoids known collectively as silymarin, is a valuable herb with a long history. The ancient Greeks recommended that its root be mixed with honey as a cough medicine. It wasn't until the sixteenth century, however, that physicians discovered that it was useful in the treatment of liver disorders.

In fact, milk thistle's real field of action appears to be the pro-

Pharmacist's Corner

■ Milk thistle is used as an injectable in Germany as the antidote for mushroom poisoning—that's how strong its liver (hepatic) protective effects are. Milk thistle is hepatoprotective at a dosage of one 175-milligram capsule three times a day with food, supplying 80% or more of silymarin per capsule.

■ Start taking this herb at low doses if you are an ex-alcoholic. I have seen alcoholics experience lower abdominal pain when they start this herb at too high a dose.

tection of the liver from various toxins, everything from alcohol to mushroom poisoning. Recent research suggests that that protection will extend to carcinogens—and not only in the liver. For example, a study on mice done at Case Western Reserve University in Cleveland showed that the number and size of skin tumors induced by UV radiation could be reduced by 67 percent and 66 percent, respectively, with administration of silymarin, milk thistle's flavonoid.

Milk thistle is known to have both antioxidant and membrane-stabilizing actions. I believe this herb has an important role to play in medicine that will fully justify its traditional uses.

CURCUMIN

Curcumin is a vigorous antioxidant and, if an increasing body of evidence is to be believed, an extremely potent anticarcinogen. Like rosemary, it is a powerful inhibitor of the COX-2 enzyme. This food ingredient is the major active component in turmeric, and turmeric is one of the major spices in curry powders. It's no surprise, therefore, that India is the largest producer and consumer of turmeric. A major spice in China and in some of the countries of the Caribbean, it is of ancient origin.

For many centuries, Indian Ayurvedic medicine has regarded turmeric as a medicinal herb effective in the treatment of gastrointestinal disorders and skin diseases. Turmeric is also an essential element in food preparation and storage because its powdered rhizome (underground stem or root) preserves freshness and nutritional value when added to food. In tropical countries, where food can rot literally within hours, this is a spice with obvious practical value.

The chemical structure of curcumin, which is one of a group of phenolic compounds present in turmeric, was first determined by Lampe in 1910. By the 1980s, with medicine now taking antioxidants seriously, extensive research on curcumin began in earnest.

With this research, the anticarcinogenic powers of curcumin have become clearer. Let's briefly consider what's been done to date:

- Curcumin has been found to be effective as a treatment for difficult cases of skin cancer. One study with genuinely startling results involved 62 patients with ulcerating cancers in their mouth or on their skin whose problems had not been adequately addressed by standard therapies—surgery, radiation, and chemotherapy. An average of 18 months of treatment with an extract of turmeric for the oral cancers and an ointment of curcumin in petroleum jelly for the skin cancers brought considerable relief from a number of unpleasant symptoms. This herbal therapy was found to have been effective in reducing the smell of the lesions (often very unpleasant) in 90 percent of the patients, reducing itching and fluid discharge from the cancerous area in 70 percent, and reducing pain and size of the lesions in 50 percent.

- C. V. Rao, Ph.D., demonstrated recently that the formation of colon tumors was inhibited in a group of rats fed curcumin.
- Another study on the influence of curcumin in the formation of breast tumors in rats also produced positive findings. The curcumin had an inhibitory effect here.
- In a study of golden hamsters, researchers found the spice itself—that is, turmeric—inhibited the formation of oral cancers induced by the application of a powerful carcinogen.
- Researchers have also found that breast and stomach tumors were inhibited by supplementation of 1 percent turmeric in rodents' daily diet.

Meanwhile, many of the methods by which carcinogensis progresses have been shown to be retarded or short-circuited by curcumin. A powerful carcinogen, TPA, is known to cause cancers partly by increasing a substance called protein kinase. Curcumin appears to suppress the production of protein kinase, as well as radically lowering levels of an oncogene, or a cancer-causing gene, called c-*jun*. A team of researchers not only demonstrated these suppressive effects but caused a 98 percent inhibition of TPA-induced tumors on mouse skin.

It is obvious that curcumin is closing off some of the cancer-causing pathways and probably blocking the formation of malignant tumors at the initiation, promotion, and progression stages of development. It is also clearly capable of actually slowing or preventing genetic mutation in cells that are at risk for cancer. Mutation is a genetic change in the DNA of a cell that gets passed on to future generations of cells in the process of cell division. Although not all mutations are carcinogenic, cancers—by definition—have followed a mutagenically altered pathway from normal cell development.

At least two studies have dramatically indicated that this pathway can be affected by curcumin. In one study, mutagenic changes in the bone marrow of mice were significantly decreased by the administration of curcumin. Another study was especially interesting because it was done on people. Obviously, for ethical reasons, human beings cannot be asked to dose themselves with carcinogens, but inveterate smokers do so quite regularly and against all warnings. In this study, then, 16 chronic smokers in India were each given approximately 1.5 grams of curcumin a day for 30 days. During that period, there was a 40 percent decrease in the urinary excretion of tobacco-related mutagens, the suspicious by-products of cell mutation. Clearly, the curcumin phenols detoxified enough carcinogens in lung tissue to cause such a reduction in the cell mutation process.

This has the appearance of a major nutritional feat. If longer studies of more smokers confirm it, curcumin will probably join green tea on the very short list of really powerful cancer preventive agents especially suitable for the needs of the nicotine addicted. Dare I imagine future smokers' bars with pots of green tea and dishes of curry at every table?

One more mechanism of protection will, I think, complete our picture of the curcumin nutritional windfall. This relates to the well-known fact that food changes radically when it's cooked— frequently for the worse as regards cancer risk. Sometimes the structure of the food breaks down and carcinogenic compounds called pyrolysates are produced. Curcumin protects food from the formation of these carcinogens. Perhaps equally important, curcumin inhibits the formation of aflatoxin, a common carcinogen that, as you may recall, is found in corn and peanuts but also grows on many other types of food if they're poorly preserved and develop mold. Putting a little curry in your lifestyle might not be a bad idea.

Pharmacist's Corner

■ Turmeric, like fish oils, inhibits the activation of the cycloxygenase-2 (COX-2) enzyme, helping to prevent the formation of PGE-2 and PGF-2D, the prostaglandins involved in inflammatory diseases and many cancers. For this reason, turmeric is great for decreasing arthritic pain and inflammation as well as helping to prevent cancer of at least the breast, colon, and prostate. Turmeric also protects the liver and has been shown in studies to help prevent cholesterol damage to blood vessel walls.

■ For its antioxidant effect, take one 300-milligram capsule of turmeric daily with food. For inflammation, take one 300-milligram capsule three times a day, also with food. The capsule should contain not less than 95% curcumin, its active constituent.

■ **Warning:** Turmeric is a spice, so patients with ulcers or inflammatory digestive tract diseases, such as colitis or Crohn's disease, may not be able to use this herb.

We've only scratched the surface of what scientists know and are beginning to find out about herbs. There is little doubt that some of these substances have powerful anticarcinogenic effects. Most of them will be tasty additions to your diet. I certainly recommend you give them a try.

Abuzz with Nutrients

Many people raise their eyebrows when I tell them that substances as exotic sounding as bee pollen, bee propolis, and royal jelly—the special nutrient of queen bees—will contribute to their health and may even help protect them from cancer. Patients have gotten used to being told to eat a healthy diet and take their vitamins. They may not balk at adding soy and a pot of green tea to their diets, but bee pollen?

Yes, it's really so. The more I do research and the longer I treat patients, the more impressed I am with how well nature provides for us. After all, we're part of it, and most of the enzymes, coenzymes, vitamins, minerals, and phytochemicals that are in the plants and animals around us are in us, too. If we were separated from nature by some wall of natural difference, it couldn't nourish us—we would be lost—but we aren't, so let's turn to the bees. They have as much right to provide us with something special for our health as anything else in the big garden that surrounds us.

THE HARVEST OF THE BUSY BEE

Bees go out to the flowering plants and collect pollen as food for the hives. They gather the sticky stuff into "baskets" on the lower parts of their legs. Commercial bee hives use pollen traps to collect the excess pollen, which there is always a great deal of. French and British researchers have reported that pollen contains 96 substances with nutritional value, including vitamins, minerals, carotenoids, enzymes, amino acids, fatty acids, bioflavonoids. Pollen has vitamin E, inositol, pyridoxine, zinc, boron, magnesium, arginine, glutamine, and various polyphenols in it. Most of these good things are discussed elsewhere in this book because of their cancer-preventive properties.

Bee pollen, therefore, is a powerful tool. It has not, however, been very well researched, compared with the other bee products I'll discuss. There was a report way back in 1948 in the *Journal of the National Cancer Institute* stating that when bee pollen was added to the diet of experimental animals, it delayed and in some cases prevented the appearance of breast cancer. Since then, silence, unless you are intrigued (and I am) by the wealth of anecdotal data from Russia and France showing that beekeepers have a very low incidence of cancer.

PROPOLIS PROTECTION

I do have more confidence in the recent evidence related to bee propolis, a waxy resin that bees gather from poplars, pines, and other trees to waterproof their hives. Propolis has been used as a food supplement in recent years. In folk medicine, its traditional use as an anti-inflammatory, antiviral, and immunostimulatory agent is well known. There is some evidence for thinking it can inhibit certain cancers.

Japanese researchers, for instance, have found that bee propolis increases the levels of natural killer cells, a type of lymphocyte that the body inevitably calls on when it has cancer cells to kill. Interest in propolis also provoked researchers at Columbia University in New York a few years ago to investigate one of its major constituents, a chemical called caffeic acid phenethyl ester (CAPE). CAPE was shown repeatedly to block tumor-promoting and carcinogen-generating oxidation processes. Dezider Grunberger, Ph.D., the scientist involved in most of these studies, also found that CAPE could cause normal cell death (apoptosis) in aberrant cell cultures and that it helps to restrict the production of the COX-2 enzyme, the proinflammation enzyme that we talked about in Chapter 3.

More recently, scientists have demonstrated that when they induced skin tumors in mice, a rather small dose of CAPE reduced the number of tumors by 24 percent and the size of the tumors by 42 percent. A much larger CAPE dose inhibited 70 percent of the tumors and decreased the average size by 74 percent.

Although clear research does not yet exist to tell us just how potently *protective* propolis will be against cancer, this is a phytonutrient that is quite clearly nutritious and immunity enhancing. I have had no hesitation about encouraging my patients—those with and without cancer—to arm-wrestle it into their diets.

THE FOOD OF QUEENS

One final bee product that is certainly highly nutritious is royal jelly. This exotic food is the nutrient that worker bees feed to the queen bee, causing her to become larger, capable of producing 2,000 eggs a day, and longer lived. With a life span of 5 to 7 years, a queen bee lives 40 times as long as the average member of her hive! Royal jelly, therefore, is a high-powered nutrient broth—for bees and even for people.

I hope I've convinced you that bee nutrients are well worth investigating. I am strongly convinced that at least one of them—bee propolis—deserves to be in any comprehensive cancer-prevention program.

Pharmacist's Corner

■ Some patients have a cross-reactivity between royal jelly and airborne allergens, resulting in allergic symptoms. Because bee pollen interacts with bee salivary gland secretions, it is a question of whether people allergic to bee venom and plant pollen will have a cross-allergy with these products.

■ Montana Naturals is a company that makes high-quality bee products. If you're not allergic to the ingredients, these are nontoxic, nutritious foods. Take the dosage shown on the label.

■ A recently published evaluation of a range of studies also claims that royal jelly at a dosage of 50 to 100 milligrams daily decreased total cholesterol levels by about 14 percent and total serum lipid levels by 10 percent.

CHAPTER 11

ALGAE, SEAWEED, AND WHEAT GRASS

*Seaweed is a delicacy fit for the most
honorable guest, even for the king himself.*

—SZE TEU (600 *B.C.*)

Unless you're Japanese, you'll probably think this chapter discusses foods you've never dreamed of eating. Swallow seaweed? Eat algae, that green pond scum stuff? Ugaa! What about wheat grass? In fact, what is it? All these foods are very basic, apparently extremely beneficial, and, in the case of algae, which sits at the bottom of the food chain, literally the earliest stuff of life. These biochemically very interesting plant foods are packed with a rich broth of nutrients. It could well be that they're the healthiest foods you haven't been eating.

Let's look at these mystery foods one by one, starting with the algae.

SPIRULINA AND CHLORELLA

Algae are the one-celled organisms that lived in the oceans and along the shores when life first began on this planet. They are still living there, tireless little food factories that convert the energy of the sun into life-giving nutrients. Many sea creatures, including the whale, subsist in whole or in part on phytoplankton, a form of algae that drift in the currents of the sea. We're going to look at two forms of algae.

First, there is spirulina, an algae that lives in bodies of warm, fresh water. When Hernánd Cortés led his 500 Spanish conquistadors into Mexico in 1518, spirulina was probably the main source of protein for the Aztecs. They gathered this blue-green algae off the surface of Lake Texcoco, where Mexico City stands today. Many historically minded biologists believe that it was the spirulina that provided a nutrient-rich topping to the Aztecs' mainly starch-based diet, giving them the raw energy they needed to build and sustain

131

a dynamic civilization. Unfortunately, after dethroning Montezuma, ravaging his capital, and expropriating his treasure, the Spaniards celebrated their conquest with a vigorous program of land reclamation—thus unwittingly destroying the nutritional basis of Indian culture!

Spirulina is 60 percent protein by weight, supplying all eight of the human body's essential amino acids. It is one of the few dietary sources of the essential fatty acid gamma-linolenic acid and has a rich supply of chlorophyll and vitamins B_{12} and B_6. It also has a phenomenal supply of carotenoids—the concentrations in spirulina are 10 times higher than in carrots.

There is also intriguing evidence that spirulina discourages the development of cancer. A 1988 study showed that spirulina (combined with another algae called dunaliella) prevented tumor development in animals given chemical carcinogens. More dramatically, a Byelorussian study found immune function enhanced in 45 children given spirulina for 45 days after the Chernobyl radiation disaster. In 83 percent of the children, a decrease in radiation activity in the urine was reported.

A recent clinical study of spirulina also gives fairly strong evidence of the algae's cancer-preventive potential. In a year-long study in which participants received either spirulina or a placebo, researchers gave one gram of freeze-dried spirulina to 60 people with premalignant lesions of the mouth, otherwise known as oral leukoplakia. The lesions completely disappeared in 44 percent of the people. Within one year after discontinuing supplemental spirulina, however, 45 percent of these people developed new lesions.

Another freshwater green algae, chlorella, may be equally sig-

Pharmacist's Corner

■ The blue-green algae spirulina is a tiny aquatic plant that is available in powder, tablet, and capsule form. Earthrise makes a very high quality spirulina product with a typical dosage of 1 heaping teaspoon mixed with fruit juice daily.

Pharmacist's Corner

■ Chlorella, a small green algae, is available from a number of manufacturers. One of my favorites is Sun Chlorella, which provides a pure and dependable product. Take 3 grams daily in juice.

nificant. It is estimated that in Japan more than five million people take it supplementally every day. It, too, is rich in chlorophyll, minerals, vitamins, and other biologically active ingredients. Incidentally, chlorophyll, the substance that makes plants green, has been shown in many studies to have anticarcinogenic effects. A study done in the 1980s on a variety of nutrients to see which would most effectively inhibit mutations caused by the chemicals in cigarette smoke gave the prize to chlorophyllin, which is the sodium-copper salt of chlorophyll. Other research has shown that chlorophyllin helps to protect deoxyribonucleic acid (DNA) from radiation damage.

A SEAWEED SELECTION

I hope to induce you to salivate over seaweed. Of course, seaweeds might be more acceptable if people would call them sea vegetables, which they really are. Under any name, they are exceedingly acceptable and beneficial fare to many peoples of the Pacific, especially the Japanese. Countless varieties of edible seaweed exist, and someday someone will write a very interesting book describing them all and explaining their nutritional qualities. They come in different colors (brown, red, and green, principally). In addition to a wide variety of essential amino acids, a bumper crop of carotenoids, and several vitamins, these seaweed veggies contain almost every mineral and trace mineral necessary for human survival. The vegetables of the sea are far richer in minerals than are most land plants.

A particularly well researched and interesting specimen is laminaria, the brown seaweed that is better known as kelp. Laminaria is high in vitamin C, chlorophyll, carotenoids, and many minerals, particularly calcium, iodine, potassium, and magnesium. In traditional medicine, kelp has been used to treat respiratory and gastrointestinal problems. Modern researchers have also discovered that it lowers blood pressure and cholesterol.

All these health benefits, however, may pale beside the significance of kelp in cancer prevention. Studies in Japan have already been done showing a direct inverse relationship between the amount of seaweed consumed and the likelihood of contracting colon or rectal cancer. Other researchers have taken substances derived from kelp and found that they protected the mucous membranes of the mouth and throat from malignant changes.

Jane Teas, Ph.D., of the Harvard School of Public Health in Boston has been in the forefront of kelp research and believes the seaweed, which is so widely consumed in Japan that estimating average daily intake is no easy matter, is significantly involved in the relative immunity Japanese women have to breast cancer.

What *is* responsible for the fact that women in Japan have one third the risk of getting breast cancer and one seventh the risk of dying of it that women in America and most northern European countries have? By this chapter, you will have noticed that we suggest several causes. Consumption of soy appears highly significant. Heavy intake of cold-water fish is a critical protective factor. Green tea consumption is probably important, too, and the lower level of fat in the Japanese diet may play a role. Now it appears that seaweed also helps. We've known for some time now that rats fed kelp have less breast cancer. T. Hirayama, M.D., has pointed out that in Japan, the lowest rates of breast cancer are in rural towns and villages, where seaweed is still consumed at almost every meal, in sauces, in salads, as vegetables and garnishes, and even mixed with the flour from which noodles are made. In Japanese cities, however, where seaweed consumption has been decreasing, breast cancer rates have been steadily rising.

I believe a good deal of kelp research still remains to be done. Nonetheless, this sea vegetable's immunity-stimulating properties, its high nutrient content, and evidence that it helps to bind pollutants already suggest a serious role for it in cancer prevention.

Pharmacist's Corner

■ Kelp is a good source of minerals, particularly iodine, which is needed for the manufacturing of thyroid hormone. If you do not get enough iodine because you do not eat fish or seafood, you avoid the salt shaker, and iodine is not in your multivitamin pill, consider a daily kelp tablet.

■ Kelp, as well as other sorts of sea vegetables, are available in health-food stores.

WHEAT, BARLEY, AND ALFALFA

Many scientists now suspect that the earth's grasses may be good for us as well as for the cows. Extracts of wheat, barley, and alfalfa are rich in flavonoid compounds that have a wide variety of beneficial effects. They have been shown to have antiviral, antitumor, and anti-inflammatory activities. One flavonoid in young green barley

Pharmacist's Corner

■ Wheat contains a type of protein called gluten that a very small group of people have difficulty in digesting, resulting in a rare disease known as celiac sprue. In these particular individuals, the gluten content can be devastating. Wheat-grass juice powder and other grass juice powders, however, are made without the protein content of the wheat. As a result, gluten-sensitive individuals can often take grass juice powders without experiencing the gastrointestinal effects of wheat. Gluten-sensitive individuals should first take extremely minimal amounts of wheat grass to determine if they have a reaction.

■ One to two teaspoons of wheat grass juice powder in your favorite juice two to three times a week is a sufficient amount of this healthy food.

leaves—glycosyl isovitexin—is one of the most powerful antioxidants yet discovered.

Chlorophyllin, the sodium-copper salt of chlorophyll that I discussed in the algae section above, is abundantly present in all grass juices and appears to inhibit a wide variety of carcinogens even at low doses. These include carcinogens in cooked meat products and in cigarette smoke.

What we call wheat grass is taken from wheat kernels harvested after seven to ten days. These young kernels are enzymatically extremely rich.

GREEN AND DESIGNER SUPERFOODS

The substances discussed in this chapter, which certainly form no part of the average American's diet, are nonetheless widely available in various green drinks sold in health-food markets. These usually contain combinations of chlorella, spirulina, wheat and barley grasses, vegetable concentrates, and other nutrients. I know that very few of you are really interested in hunting out sources of seaweed and algae to put in your daily menu. Therefore, I recommend that you find yourself a good green drink or a green powder that can be mixed with water, tea, or some other beverage of your choice.

The kind of drink I recommend should have a content list that is somewhat similar to the ingredients you'll find in the box on pages 138–139. Drinks like this are very high powered nutritional tools, and not only will they offer you a variety of cancer protective phytonutrients, but they will provide you with a lot of energy, too. I invariably press them on my patients, who, after a period of adjustment, generally report great satisfaction with their new energy levels.

Pharmacist's Corner

■ Not all green designer foods are created equally. Many times, the central ingredient is soybean powder, the least expensive ingredient and, in this form, physiologically acidifying—not a very healthy choice. A good portion of these products are also given to healthy bacterial cultures, initially a good idea, although it is questionable whether these cultures will survive in the mixture of herbs offered, especially when stocked unrefrigerated on store shelves. Typically, the contents are healthy but the more expensive ingredients, alas, are left by the wayside. Be wary of products that do not give the number in milligrams of each ingredient on the label; this may mean there is very little of the ingredient in the product and the milligram content is low.

■ A good designer food includes a high concentration of flaxseed meal, which supplies omega-3 fatty acids, a good quantity of esoteric healthy nutrients (such as propolis, royal jelly, high-pectin apple fiber, and rosemary), and a mixture of herbs, phytochemicals, algaes, grass juice powders, glutathione promoters, amino acids, and vitamins.

Suggested Contents of a Superior Green Drink

Serving size: 9.69 grams; servings per container: 45

Contents of 3 Heaping Scoops (milligrams)	% Daily Value
Phytonutrients	
High-pectin apple fiber, 1,350	*
Soy lecithin, 4,250	*
Brown rice germ, 700	*
Royal jelly, 1,000	*
Bee propolis, 2,400	*
Acerola berry juice powder, 230	*
Grape skin, 300	*
Carrot juice, 500	*
Flaxseed meal, 4,000	*
Bee pollen, 1,000	*
Red clover, 60	*
Burdock root, 60	*
Dandelion, 60	*
Parsley, 60	*
Rose hips, 60	*
Ginger, 160	*
Siberian ginseng, 60	*
Rosemary, 60	*
Curcumin, 60	*
Grapefruit seed extract, 25	*
Spinach, 100	*
Broccoli, 100	*
Guaranteed-potency herbs and phytochemicals	
Grape seed extract, 40 (standardized to 95% polyphenols)	*
Japanese green tea, 40 (standardized to 7.5% catechins, predominantly as epigallocatechin gallate [EGCG])	*
Soy isoflavones, 750 (supplying 12–14 milligrams of genistein, genistin, daidzin, daidzein, glycitin, and glycitein)	*
Bilberry (European), 20 (standarized to 25% anthocyanocides)	*
Ginkgo biloba, 60 (standarized to 24% ginkgoflavonglycosides and 6% terpenes)	*

Lycopene, 10   *
Garlic (odorless), Puregar, 250 (1,500 parts per million   *
    allicin yield)
Milk thistle, 120 (standarized to 80% silymarin)   *

Alpha amino acids
    L-carnitine, 250   *
    L-glutamine, 250   *
    L-arginine, 250   *

Algae (blue and green)
    Spirulina, 1,300   *
    Blue-green algae (Klamath Lake), 1,500   *
    CGC Chlorella, broken cell, 350   *
    Digitata kelp, 40   *
    Irish moss, 40   *

Green grass juice powders
    Barley grass, 1,350   *
    Oat grass, 1,350   *
    Wheat grass, 1,350   *
    Alfalfa grass, 1,350   *

Other nutrients
    N-acetyl-L-cysteine, 600   *
    Alpha-lipoic acid, 100   *

B-complex vitamins
    Thiamine HC (vitamin B_1), 50   3,333
    Riboflavin (vitamin B_2), 50   2,941
    Pyridoxine HC (vitamin B_6), 50   2,500
    Niacinamide, 100   500
    Pantothenic acid, 250   2,500
    Vitamin B_{12}, 250 micrograms   4,167
    PABA (para-aminobenzoic acid), 50   *
    Biotin, 100 micrograms   33
    Folic acid, 400 micrograms   100
    Choline bitartrate, 100   *
    Inositol, 100   *

Mild natural licorice flavor

*Daily value not established.

CHAPTER 12

MUSHROOMS AND IMMUNITY

The Chinese do not draw any distinction between food and medicine.

—LIN YUTANG

In China alone, there are more than 270 different varieties of mushrooms in use for medical treatment, and a fair number of these are believed to possess anticarcinogenic properties. Mushroom enthusiasm in China, intermingled with Taoist philosophy, has led to the concept that mushrooms boost *chi* or life energy. The Japanese, almost as mushroom crazy as their neighbors, not only believe that this strange form of higher fungi may be, as a seventeenth-century medical scholar said, the "elixir of life" but have made it into an important part of their culture and nutritional tradition. They spend more than $2 billion a year on this culinary delight.

By actively researching the chemical properties of mushrooms, they have discovered that there is plenty of scientific backup for the medical traditions of the Orient. The evidence—by this time, there is a good deal of it—leads me to think that mushrooms ought to be at the cutting edge of cancer prevention. Certainly, they ought to be in your diet, especially if you can afford some of the more exotic Asian mushrooms such as maitake, shiitake, and reishi.

THE DANCING MUSHROOM

Maitake (botanical name: *Grifola frondosa*) will be the leading fungi in this chapter. Supposedly its Japanese nickname, "the dancing mushroom," came about because back in the days when all peasants were poor, anyone so fortunate as to come across one on the hillsides of northeastern Japan would start to dance for joy—these hefty mushrooms (some clusters of maitake weigh in at 100 pounds) sold for vast sums in the marketplace.

Extremely sensitive to environmental changes, maitake remained rare until recent years, when the Japanese developed methods of cultivating it. Now you can get it in high-quality grocery stores and health-food stores (at a high price) in North America. It is not only a delicious food but the possessor of chemical properties that almost any cancer would find discouraging.

The initial research on this mushroom was done by Japanese scientist Hiroaki Nanba, Ph.D. He showed that maitake not only stimulates immune function but inhibits tumor growth. The crucial compounds in this big mountain mushroom are polysaccharides; one polysaccharide in particular, beta-glucan, is a formidable cancer antagonist.

In 1986, Dr. Nanba conducted an experiment on mice injected with tumor cells. Some of the mice were given feed, of which 20 percent was powdered maitake mushroom. Another group was given powdered shiitake mushroom. The shiitake group had a 77.9 percent inhibition of tumor growth; the maitake group, an 86.3 percent inhibition. This was formidable interference in the cancer process, and this initial study prompted many others.

The mushrooms were on the march. It seems quite clear that much of the tumor inhibition effect was caused by immune system stimulation. Back in the early days of cancer investigation, it was assumed that cancer cells were relatively rare malfunctions of the body and that the reason most of us didn't die of cancer was because the process that leads to a full-grown malignancy never got started. We have long since learned better. You'll remember that the average cell takes 10,000 free-radical hits on its deoxyribonucleic acid (DNA) daily, and you have trillions of cells. Rogue cancer cells are commonplace; but your body is designed to deal with them.

One of the ways it does so is with the vigorous, vigilant, and deadly armed forces at its command. Scientists have given various colorful names to these molecular assassins—natural killer cells, for instance. Among their many duties are sensing other cells that are dividing at an abnormally rapid rate—which is, of course, characteristic of cancers—and traveling to the site of the improper activity to deliver a killing dose of chemical toxicity. It is by such swift and unappealable justice that most of the cancer cells in your body end up as molecular corpses not so very long after their creation. In other words, your own body does most of the work of stopping cancer. Why not help it along?

This and other questions prompted Nanba and his colleagues to conduct their next mouse study with maitake. They reported that the mushroom "directly activates various effector cells (macrophages, natural killer cells, killer T-cells, etc.) to attack tumor cells."

Researchers at the National Cancer Institute, a division of the National Institutes of Health in Bethesda, Maryland, were also intrigued by maitake and discovered that maitake extract was active against the acquired immunodeficiency syndrome (AIDS) virus as well. It appeared that the polysaccharide compounds in the mushroom helped to stop the virus from killing T-cells. These, too, are vitally important members of your immune system army, trained to recognize and attack bacterial and viral enemies.

The fact that maitake is apparently the most powerful immune system stimulant and cancer fighter among the Oriental mushrooms is interesting because three different anticancer drugs have already been extracted from other mushrooms and approved by the Japanese Health and Welfare Ministry (the equivalent of the U.S. Food and Drug Administration [FDA]). These are lentinan, derived from shiitake; schizophyllan, derived from suehirotake; and PSK, derived from kawaratake. PSK, widely sold in Europe and Japan, is, by some accounts, the best-selling cancer drug in the world. All the evidence seems to show that although PSK certainly cannot handle cancer on its own, it does provide effective support to chemotherapeutic regimens.

In all investigations of the effects of various mushrooms on cancer conducted in animals so far, maitake, however, has proven most effective. Why? Another Japanese researcher, Kyoko Adachi, has studied the actions of beta-glucan (the major maitake polysaccharide) when given to counter tumors in mice. He concluded that this polysaccharide not only activates the strongarm members of the mammalian immune system—macrophages, natural killer cells, and killer T-cells—but also potentiates (makes possible) the activity of various mediators of immune system activity, such as lymphokines and interleukin-1. Interleukin-1 causes the cells to produce interleukin-2, which in turn causes T-cells to rapidly increase. In fact, interleukin-2 has been called T-cell growth factor. What the Japanese believe they have demonstrated is that the polysaccharides in maitake mushrooms provide a complete program of immune system stimulation that can quite adequately explain the potency of their effects on cancer.

MORE MAITAKE

In 1995, Dr. Nanba published yet another extremely impressive animal study of maitake involving three groups of mice. The first group was given a typical mouse diet, a control diet. The second group was given a diet containing 20 percent maitake powder. The third group was given an oral dose of maitake extract at the rate of 1 milligram per kilogram of body weight. Then all the mice were given a carcinogen three times at 7-day intervals. Two months later, liver tumors were counted. Let's take the results in reverse order. In the third group (given the maitake extract), liver cancer occurred in 9.7 percent of the mice. In the second group (given the maitake powder diet), malignancies occurred in 22.2 percent. The first group—the poor little mice without maitake—weren't so lucky. One hundred percent of them developed cancer. It was an impressive instance of cancer prevention.

Another study by Nanba has compared maitake extract (called D-fraction) with a widely used chemotherapeutic agent called mitomycin-C. A relatively small dose of the maitake extract produced an 80 percent tumor regression, compared with 30 percent when mitomycin-C alone was used. When combined together, the two shrunk the mouse tumors by 98 percent, an obviously impressive syngeristic effect.

Speaking at the Adjuvant Nutrition in Cancer Treatment Symposium in Tampa, Florida, in October 1995, Dr. Nanba described the effects of maitake extract given in conjunction with standard chemotherapy to 165 patients with advanced cancer. Severe side effects appear to have been ameliorated by this treatment. In interpreting the results of this sort of uncontrolled study, however, I am always more cautious, for it is difficult to measure success here.

Dr. Nanba's own closing observations on the effectiveness of the treatment were as follows: "Though it cannot be said that mai-take D-fraction [considered to be the most active constituent in this mushroom] and tablets are the cancer cure, one can safely say that they do maintain the quality of life of patients and improve the immune system, resulting in the possible remission of cancer cells with no side effects." I am hoping that further research will show that this fairly optimistic position has merit.

NOT JUST MAITAKE

Meanwhile, there continues to exist the possibility that the other Oriental mushrooms will eventually play an important role. Certainly, at the least, they are highly nutritious. Ounce for ounce, shiitake, the large, meaty, exquisitely flavorful black mushroom that has established a firm footing in the gourmet grocery stores of America, has twice the protein and fiber of the typical supermarket mushroom. It also has far more calcium and high levels of the B vitamins and vitamin D_2. Whatever its effects on cancer, well-conducted studies seem to show that it drops cholesterol and lowers blood pressure. It has been part of the traditional medicine of Asia for thousands of years.

A major component in shiitake (botanical name: *Lentinus edodes*) is the polysaccharide lentinan. Like maitake's polysaccharides, lentinan has been shown to boost interleukin-1 levels and to increase the cytotoxic (cell-destroying) activity of macrophages.

Pharmacist's Corner

■ Maitake mushroom contains a substance referred to as D-fraction or Special-Fraction. The dosage for stimulating the immune system is two capsules two times daily in between meals supplying a total of 12 milligrams of D-fraction.

■ Maitake mushroom tea bags are available. A cup two to four times a day is nowhere as strong as taking the capsules but a sip in the right direction.

Pharmacist's Corner

■ Shiitake mushrooms taste wonderful and are a delicious addition to dishes if cut up and used as a seasoning. Try shiitake mushroom as an appetizer by preparing it with garlic, parsley, basil, and a little olive oil, then baking it until it's tender. Use as much or as little as you wish.

■ If you detest the taste of mushrooms, try taking a shiitake extract 600-milligram capsule twice daily, which supplies 6 milligrams of the KS-2 polysaccharides.

There have been reports that scientists at Semmelweis Medical University in Budapest, Hungary, have found that lentinan can modify cells so that they resist the metastasis of lung cancer cells. Finally, like maitake but to a lesser extent, shiitake has inhibited mouse tumors.

The third mushroom powerhouse from Asia is reishi (botanical name: *Ganoderma lucidum*). It has its own set of polysaccharides, as well as a long traditional history of use in Chinese medicine. Chinese herbalists believed that it benefits the heart, and in the 1980s, Japanese researchers confirmed that it did indeed lower

Pharmacist's Corner

■ Reishi mushroom tea tastes delicious. I brew and drink a mixture of reishi mushroom, red clover, burdock root, and green tea two to three times daily to support my immune function, flood my system with antioxidants, and help my body to detoxify.

■ Reishi mushrooms are available in 420-milligram capsules and nonalcoholic tincture. The dosage would typically be 1 or 2 capsules three times a day. The tincture dosage is 10 drops three times daily in juice.

blood pressure in patients with hypertension as well as lower cholesterol and triglyceride levels.

On the cancer front, more reishi research is necessary. There have been intriguing but unconfirmed reports of its positive effects in cancer patients. Certainly, the studies that have been done so far seem to show that like its fungal cousins, maitake and shiitake, it has immunostimulating powers. It is believed to increase the output of macrophages and T-cells, and it has been successfully used in the treatment of viral hepatitis.

The bottom line on mushrooms—especially maitake—is that their cancer-preventive effects are certainly real. Could their therapeutic effects in the treatment of cancer be real as well? More research is desperately needed. Eventually, scientists will explore and explain the full potential of these marvelous fungi, but for now, we can be sure that Oriental mushrooms are nutritious, delicious, and possibly tumoricidal. Mushrooms are an old, old life-form, first appearing in Asia around 100 million years ago. I suspect that you, too, would like to become a fairly old life-form—so eat your mushrooms.

CHAPTER 13

SHARKS, OLIVES, AND OTHER GOOD THINGS

Life is not living, but living in health.

—MARTIAL

SHARKS

Sharks—even apart from their teeth—are among the most fascinating creatures on earth. They are a 200 million-year-old success story that were chewing and swallowing with gustatory enthusiasm long before we discovered our first cave. Found in all the ocean waters of the earth from the Arctic to the Antarctic, they are protected not only by their formidable dental showpieces but by an immune system that is second to nothing on the planet. Why does the average shark live to advanced old age—in some cases close to 100 years? Why are sharks able to heal wounds caused by other sharks with astonishing rapidity? Why don't sharks get cancer?

Many scientists now believe that if you want the answer, you should look into the shark's liver. This gigantic organ frequently comprises more than 20 percent of the predator's size and weight. The shark's liver contains exceptionally high levels of two important natural compounds: alkylglycerol (AKG) and squalene. Those substances are the subject of this chapter.

ALKYLGLYCEROLS AND THE IMMUNE SYSTEM

AKGs are fats that are present in human and cow's milk and in the bone marrow, spleen, and liver of most animals and fishes. It has been proven that AKGs vigorously stimulate immune function. They are considered to be one of the main reasons that human breast milk (which incidentally has 10 times the amount of AKGs found in cow's milk) is so important to the development of an optimally functioning immune system in infants.

AKGs were first discovered in 1922 by Japanese researchers dissecting sharks caught in the deep waters off New Zealand. In the

153

1950s, Swedish doctor Astrid Brohult noticed the positive effect on children hospitalized with leukemia of a substance taken from the bone marrow of calves. Although it took years to determine, the active ingredient turned out to be AKGs. Working with a Swedish pharmaceutical company, Dr. Brohult and her husband, Sven Brohult, a professor of chemistry, started looking for a source of AKGs and discovered that in the Atlantic Ocean, there was simply no source better than the oil that comes from the liver of the Greenland shark. AKGs were tremendously abundant in shark liver oil, and the Greenland shark, a relatively benign deep-water fish, had a lot of liver. They found, as so often is the case, that what was new to science was not new to humankind. Northern fishermen had been using shark liver oil as a home remedy and health-enhancing agent for generations.

Shark liver oil activates the whole immune system team, including leukocytes, lymphocytes, and macrophages, a motley crew of warrior cells that really have it in for cancers. Since, pound for pound, sharks have more AKGs than does any other living creature, this may well be a thoroughly adequate explanation for their near-perfect immunity from cancer. In human breast milk, one tenth of 1 percent of the fat content of the milk is AKGs. In shark liver oil, anywhere from 10 percent to 30 percent of the fat is AKGs. That's a concentration 100 to 300 times as great, yet, human breast milk is a high-quality immunity-enhancing drink. No baby should leave home without it.

Pharmacist's Corner

■ Oceana™ is the trade name for a high quality shark liver oil product. Oceana™ is a 570-milligram capsule supplying 125 milligrams of alkoxyglycerols and 110 milligrams squalene per capsule. A starting dosage is one capsule three times daily with meals for two weeks then reduce it to one capsule two times daily with food.

SHARK LIVER OIL AGAINST TUMORS

By the early 1970s, it had already been demonstrated that shark liver oil could inhibit the growth of tumors in experimental animals. Human studies have focused on giving shark liver oil as an addition and in conjunction with conventional therapies, with extremely positive results. Patients with cervical cancer who received AKGs at the time they were receiving radiotherapy had significantly reduced the injuries resulting from radiation toxicity and showed an increased survival rate; among those who eventually did not live, there was a longer survival time. Research by Dr. Astrid Brohult on patients with the same disease turned up very similar results. Patients were given AKGs for seven days before treatment with radiation; a reduced percentage of these patients went on to advanced stages of the tumor. In effect, there was tumor regression in some patients. Dr. Brohult also did a study of such patients showing a reduction in the number of patients who died, with remarkably higher survival rates among women who were younger than 60 years old.

I believe AKGs are a vast field awaiting exploration. Since this is a book primarily about cancer prevention, not cancer treatment, I hope the above studies will not apply to any of my readers. What does apply to everyone are the demonstrated immune system enhancements produced by AKGs, one of the main components of shark liver oil. You, too, have AKGs in your body, but I think you might consider increasing their number supplementally.

SQUALENE: SHARED BY SHARKS AND OLIVES

What, I'm sure you'd like to know, does the humble and beneficient olive have in common with the ferocious shark? Nothing much, apart from uniquely high levels of a substance called squalene. You've probably never heard of squalene before, but whether you make olive oil or shark liver oil your beverage of choice, you will go away from the encounter nutritionally richer for your consumption of this pleasantly bland tasing hydrocarbon contained in both oils.

Let's turn away from squalene, though, for just one moment. The really interesting direction from which to approach this whole

The Shark Cartilage Story

Many of you will remember the hoopla surrounding shark cartilage several years ago. It was reported on a TV broadcast early in 1994 in a segment on *60 Minutes* that the cartilage in sharks (sharks have no skeleton, so we certainly can't investigate their bone marrow) could reverse cancer by reversing angiogenesis, the process whereby a cancer builds up its own special blood vessel system to supply itself with nutrients. A clinical trial in Cuba seemed to show greatly increased survival rates among patients with terminal cancer who had been given shark cartilage.

After other news media repeated the story, sales of the substance soared in health-food stores, and new hope was given to many. Unfortunately, attempts to reproduce the results reported in Cuba have not met with success. It looked as if shark cartilage was doomed to be nothing more than a footnote in the history of fads.

In the spring of 1998, however, a new development occurred. Gerald Batiste, M.D., of the prestigious McGill University in Montreal, Quebec, Canada, presented a report to the American Association for Cancer Research on work that he and his research team had done with an extract from shark cartilage called AE-941. They divided patients with advanced tumors of the prostate, breast, and lung among four groups of five to six patients each and gave each group a different dose of AE-941. Dr. Batiste reported that blood vessel growth around the tumors was blocked and that tumor growth was checked, with patients taking the highest dose of the extract showing the greatest response.

Batiste's team conducted a further trial of AE-941 with 30 patients, each of whom was given the highest dose of the extract. The results of this trial have just been released with very favorable indications.

Then in September 1998, the National Cancer Institute, National Institutes of Health, took a major step toward cancer prevention. Liquid shark cartilage AE-941 was approved for Phase III Clinical Trials, specifically to evaluate its efficacy in the treatment of cancer. Pending regulatory review, the trials are scheduled for early 1999. They include a multicenter Phase III double-blind placebo-controlled trial in which the liquid shark cartilage will be given to several hundred cancer patients in hospitals and institutions across the United States.

This is an important validation of the use of liquid shark cartilage and I eagerly await the results from this clinical trial.

Incidentally, the new drug developed in Boston by Judah Folkmann, PhD., and his team and so widely discussed in the press, works on the same principle: prevention of new blood vessel growth. There is, by now, a history of drugs that made cancers go away in mice and couldn't perform the same feat in people. To date, Dr. Folkmann's antiangiogenesis pharmaceuticals have been tested only on mice and whether the big step from mice to humans can be done remains to be seen.

CarTCell by Allergy Research Group is a liquid shark cartilage supplement, manufactured by the producers of AE-941. It is sold in nutritional pharmacies and is listed in the Resource Section. For more information call Allergy Research Group at **800-545-9960.**

subject is to ask why a high consumption of olive oil is associated with a sharp drop in levels of breast cancer and probably several other types of cancer. In Greece, women take approximately 40 percent of their caloric intake from fat. That was the level American women were at until a slight decline in recent years. Contrary to any simplistic theory about the relationship of fat consumption to breast cancer, however, Greek women have only one-third the incidence of breast cancer of American women. That isn't the end of the good news for Greek women. Those among them who consume olive oil more than once a day have a further reduction of 25 percent of their breast cancer risk. This phenomenon is not confined to Greece. Most of the major olive oil–consuming countries surrounding the Mediterranean show a similar pattern. A study done in Spain showed a reduced breast cancer risk in women consuming the most olive oil. Similar research in Italy suggests that olive oil exerts protective effects; the edible oil consumed by Italians is olive oil about 80 percent of the time. An Italian study done in 1990 also showed decreased incidence of pancreatic cancer in people who consumed the most olive oil.

The protective effect of olive oil had been thought to be due to the high proportion of it (72 percent) that comes from the monounsaturated fatty acid oleic acid. This fatty acid is also found in beef and poultry (45 percent of fat) as well as in other vegetable oils, such as corn, palm, soybean, and sunflower seed. And many of these other fats and oils rich in oleic acid have actually shown an association with greater risk of cancer. This has caused scientists to look at squalene. Nearly 1 percent of the content of olive oil is squalene. That's a uniquely high concentration compared to what is found in the other fats and oils that human beings commonly consume. In fact, food regulatory parameters use squalene concentration to determine the purity of olive oil.

That squalene should be the good guy really doesn't come as a surprise. Studies have shown that this nutritional precursor has anticarcinogenic effects for which we seem to have a very good explanation. It inhibits skin cancers in laboratory animals caused by the potent carcinogen benzoprene. In other research, animals were protected from breast cancer, and it may be that we know the mechanism of this protection. Squalene has been found to inhibit (by 80 percent!) an enzyme called HMGcoA-reductase that—after various chemical conversions—makes possible the activation of the *ras* oncogene.

Oncogenes, by the way, are rather special genes that generally remain latent, or unactivated, throughout our lives. They never cause us problems unless they are activated, and then they will tend to push you strongly toward cancer.

The *ras* oncogene is quite an infamous culprit in cancer studies. It has been shown to have an association with many types of cancers, including melanoma, colon, breast, and pancreas. If squalene protects us, as it seems to, this may be why. Please note: the average squalene intake in the United States is only 30 milligrams a day. In Greece and Italy, with their vastly higher olive oil consumption, squalene intake is usually in the range of 200 to 400 milligrams a day.

All of this evidence points a finger squarely at squalene. There are very good logical reasons suggesting that it should be protective against cancer. Animal studies and human population studies from countries that border the Mediterranean are giving strong indications that this hypothetical protection is very real.

Pharmacist's Corner

■ Squalene is available in olive oil, but it is also available in 450-milligram capsules. One or 2 capsules daily with food will give you a sufficient supply of squalene.

I can recommend only two steps. First, incorporate olive oil in your diet. Learn to cook with it. It is by far the healthiest cooking oil in common use. Once you grow accustomed to it, start using it on your salads. In our household, we use nothing but. I suggest you use virgin or extra virgin olive oil, as these are made from the first pressings of the olive and are nutritionally richer.

My second recommendation, based on all the evidence in this chapter, is that you add shark liver oil to your list of nutritional supplements. The combination of AKGs and extra squalene that it will put in your diet will be formidably health enhancing.

CHAPTER 14

AMINO ACIDS "Я" Us

*In treating a patient, let your first thought
be to strengthen his natural vitality.*

—RHAZES

It is the amino acid units of protein that form the structure of all living things, from the tiniest microbe to the brain of Einstein. These large molecules make up 20 percent of our body weight, forming the primary components of our muscles, skin, eyes, nails, hair, and internal organs—including the heart and brain. In short, we are rich in amino acids, and we need to be.

There are 20 major amino acids, and 8 of them are regarded as essential, meaning that we must obtain them in our diet. The other 12 are just as necessary for good health but are called nonessential because if we don't eat them, our bodies will manufacture them from other substances. All of these amino acids, therefore, are necessary for life. A protein food source is only spoken of as "complete" when it contains all of them.

I could certainly write a very long chapter on the importance of the amino acids for general health, but this will be a very brief chapter concentrating on just two amino acids: arginine and glutamine. There is some very suggestive evidence that they offer protection against cancer. In our society's protein-rich diet, a shortage of amino acids is not usually a problem, except sometimes in the elderly. Therefore, in this chapter, we will consider whether there is any advantage in possessing these two amino acids at levels well above deficiency states. Indeed, the question we will have to ask ourselves is whether arginine and glutamine are appropriate for supplementation as prophylactics against cancer.

ARGININE

Arginine, which has found notoriety and popularity among body builders, is a really versatile amino acid. Here are just a few of its capacities when taken supplementally at various levels: it can enhance male fertility, detoxify harmful substances, improve the healing of wounds and burns, build muscle, increase immune function, and fight cancer.

Arginine's popularity among body builders arises from its apparent effects on human growth hormone, one of the body's principal hormones for repairing and rebuilding tissue. In studies of older people, supplemental growth hormone has been found to increase muscle mass and decrease fat, even without additional exercise. Also, growth hormone is a major repair hormone in the human body and may even offer some protection against Alzheimer's disease. Since the body's levels of growth hormone decline fairly drastically with age, hormone supplementation for the aged has been discussed as a method of bringing them back to a more youthful and healthy norm. This remains a matter of great controversy.

Whether body builders, who are mostly young people, can add

How Much Arginine and How to Get It

Arginine is richly supplied in peanuts, peanut butter, almonds, cashews, pecans, and chocolate. (Remember, however, that I don't recommend peanuts or peanut butter because of the possibility of aflatoxin contamination.) It is more moderately represented in peas, garlic, and ginseng.

The truth is, however, that although some of these are excellent foods that we recommend elsewhere, the likelihood of significantly altering your levels of arginine through dietary changes is not great.

Any serious approach to increasing arginine will probably have to involve supplementation, a topic of some controversy. Be that as it may, arginine, generally available in 500-milligram capsules, is sometimes taken in doses as high as 4 to 6 grams daily. Although many people can tolerate these levels, there are occasionally side effects, such as nausea and diarrhea. A more moderate level—2 grams or less—seems to be safe and side-effect free. Many researchers agree, however, that optimal growth hormone regulation may require at least 3 grams daily.

You should not take arginine if you have liver or kidney disorders, or if you have an active herpes infection, unless you receive the okay from your physician. Indeed, I do not advise supplementation with amino acids except under the guidance of a physician.

Pharmacist's Corner

■ L-arginine is considered conditionally essential, meaning that under conditions of extreme physical stress, we are not making enough L-arginine. As a result, additional L-arginine is required from food or supplements. Conditions in which additional L-arginine is beneficial and even lifesaving include severe infections; recuperation from major surgery; ischemic heart disease; healing wounds and burns; retention of muscle mass in endurance athletes, dieters, and the ill; and, of course, aiding a poorly functioning immune system.

■ There is anecdotal evidence that L-arginine may stimulate a herpes outbreak in people who have herpes, although there is no scientific proof for this.

■ L-arginine controls the release of nitric oxide, a neurotransmitter that is beneficial in patients with heart disease, asthma, and men with erectile dysfunction.

■ A typical dosage is 500 milligrams one to three times daily.

---

muscle by increasing growth hormone (either directly or through arginine supplementation) is highly questionable. After all, they already have an ample supply.

Many scientists believe, however, that arginine's effects on growth hormone levels may be responsible for at least part of its benefits in wound healing and enhanced immune function. Growth hormone is influential in both those areas. Research in animals has shown that the thymus gland, an important part of the immune system because it is the source of the lymphocytes that are so critical to immunity—and an area of the body that shrinks radically with age—enlarges and becomes more active after arginine supplementation. The same phenomenon has also been demonstrated in animals treated with growth hormone. Even in humans, a study of women with low growth hormone levels demonstrated that upon supplementation with the hormone, the women's natural killer cell activity increased by almost 20 percent.

It would seem likely that arginine's capacity for boosting immunity is related to its cancer-fighting and wound-healing abilities. Japanese scientists have shown in an interesting test-tube experiment that immune cells from healthy humans put together with arginine show a threefold increase in natural killer cell activity and demonstrate direct antitumor cell effects.

Such intriguing evidence has begun to prompt research in humans. A study conducted by British surgeons on 18 patients about to undergo colorectal surgery showed that administration of arginine for 3 days before surgery increased the degree to which a type of cancer-fighting cell called a tumor-infiltrating lymphocyte entered into the cells of the tumor. The ability of arginine to increase the intensity of effective attack against tumor cells in this manner has enormous implications.

Researchers are also investigating animals' responses to arginine. In a powerful study coming out of Queens University of Belfast, Ireland, a group of male rats were given a carcinogen that causes colorectal cancer. Then arginine was given to some of the rats. There was a significant reduction in tumor incidence and tumor size in the arginine-supplemented rats. It was also found—another excellent response—that lymphocyte production from the thymus had increased in the rats given arginine. This report does not stand alone; there have been more than two dozen studies in animals showing regression of tumors, slowing of tumor growth, and reduced tumor incidence in response to arginine.

I am well aware that these studies seem to suggest that arginine may eventually evolve as a part of cancer treatment. Nonetheless, its value in prevention seems undeniable. Anything that enhances the functioning of the thymus is almost certainly improving your body's defenses against malignant cells, and a substance that improves lymphocyte attack on those cells is definitely improving your capacity for cancer prevention, since, as I emphasized previously, the body produces cancer cells with terrible regularity.

GLUTAMINE

Glutamine has an interesting and somewhat mysterious relationship to cancer, and it is certainly not clear at this time whether it will prove to be as significant a cancer preventive as many of the other nutrients I've discussed. It is hardly an antagonist of cancer in any normal sense, since a tumor requires enormous amounts of glutamine to grow efficiently; without the presence of this amino acid, a cancer simply cannot prosper. That is not necessarily an indictment of glutamine, though, since without it, you would not prosper either.

Glutamine is the most abundant amino acid in blood and cerebrospinal fluid and is the only amino acid that easily passes the blood–brain barrier. It is essential to the formation of muscle, and a shortage of glutamine can lead to physical wasting. Glutamine has achieved a certain amount of notoriety because of its ability to decrease the craving for alcohol. In this regard, it is now commonly used in alcoholism clinics. It also seems that glutamine may reduce the desire for sugar and carbohydrates and it could have a role to play in controlling obesity.

The importance of glutamine in cancer prevention would seem to lie in its ability to increase natural killer cell activity. This has been demonstrated in a number of studies that have also shown that glutamine inhibits the formation of prostaglandin E_2 (PGE$_2$), which as you may remember from Chapter 7 is the prostaglandin that promotes inflammatory activity and tumor formation.

Pharmacist's Corner

■ L-glutamine is available in 500-milligram capsules, the dosage varies according to the indication. For athletes and dieters, L-glutamine donates nitrogen to the muscle and will help prevent a loss of muscle. Four 500-milligram L-glutamine capsules once daily between meals seems to be the dosage required to maintain muscle in these circumstances.

■ L-glutamine is also a major precursor for glutathione. A dosage of 1,000-milligrams once daily between meals will help maintain adequate levels of this important liver-protecting nutrient.

At this juncture, let's turn to Susan Klimberg, Ph.D., and her team of researchers at the University of Arkansas in Fayetteville. They performed an experiment on two groups of rats that they gave breast tumors to go through the implantation of tumor cells. They then fed glutamine to one group only. After 7 weeks, they killed the rats and examined them. The difference between the two groups was remarkable. Tumor growth in the glutamine-fed rats was approximately 40 percent less than in the other group. Moreover, the rate of natural killer cell activity in the glutamine rats was 2.5 times that of the rats who went without. Another method by which glutamine may control tumor growth is indicated by the fact that the rate of PGE-2 synthesis in the glutamine fed rats was 25 percent lower than in the other rats. To increase natural killer cell activity while restricting the creation of PGE-2 seems a worthwhile and even formidable cancer preventive approach.

Clearly, more studies will need to be done on glutamine's protective capacities. Two rather interesting studies have indicated how this powerful amino acid may help to mitigate some of the difficulties of cancer management and treatment.

A very interesting study from Italy has demonstrated that glutamine repairs damaged intestinal mucosa in patients who were being given chemotherapy and reduces the severity and duration of diarrhea. The dose level was very high: 18 grams a day. (In healthy patients receiving glutamine supplementation, recommended levels are seldom more than 2 grams a day.) Since anything that can mitigate the rigors of chemotherapy is pure gold, this approach needs to be studied intensively as well.

Finally, some doctors are evolving an interesting approach based on the well-known need for and appetite for glutamine shown by cancers. Researchers have noticed that a malignant tumor functions as a sort of glutamine trap, which ultimately causes glutamine depletion throughout the rest of the body. Since glutamine is vital to the formation of muscle, this depletion may be one of the principal causes of the profound weight loss and muscle wasting—the cachexia—characteristic of patients in the advanced stages of cancer. Repeated studies have begun to show that when high doses of glutamine are given to cancer patients, this may replace the glutamine the cancer has captured and may be beneficial to the patient as a means of arresting cachexia.

I am very optimistic about glutamine's future use in cancer treatment and prevention, but it is too early to make a recommendation that healthy individuals consume it supplementally as a preventive.

CHAPTER 15

VITAMINS

*But if I want to use these substances or
natural preventive agents to reduce
oxidative damage to my cells and tissues,
then I believe I need to use them in
supplemental form to achieve the
necessary dosages.*

—ANDREW WEIL, M.D.

By the end of the twentieth century, it has become very clear that vitamins will give you substantial protection from cancer. If you can get your vitamins in sufficient quantities from your food, then congratulations—you're part of a remarkable minority; if you can't, then I strongly advise a reasonable and moderate program of nutritional supplementation. No controversy should attach to such a recommendation. The evidence from clinical trials, from large-scale epidemiologic studies, and from other assorted scientific research projects is powerful and about as consistent as one can ever expect anything to be in a world as complicated as ours.

As you'll see when you read Chapter 20, "The Complete Cancer Prevention Program," I always tell my patients that they should eat an amazing variety of foods each and every day. When they come back and tell me, "That's impossible. I just don't have the time," then I say, "Okay, we'll put together the best plan that's possible for you and add a modest supplementation program to fill in the gaps."

I take vitamins and mineral supplements and so does everyone in my family. Food is best, but vitamins are a nice accessory that in the long run may make the difference between living without cancer and living (or not living) with it.

Now, let's look at the big picture before we turn to the major vitamins.

IRREPLACEABLE UNITS OF HEALTH

Vitamins are organic nutrients needed by the body for normal physiologic and metabolic functioning and well-being. The quantities of vitamins that any of us consume are small by weight compared to the total amount of food we swallow, but those small quantities are essential to good health. Without them, critical bodily processes quickly come grinding to a halt. In fact, you only have to stop eating fruits and vegetables for 1 to 2 weeks, and you will begin to notice the start of a profound physically based depression.

Vitamins must be obtained through diet. Although the skin can make some vitamin D by reacting with sunlight and the bacteria in our intestines are capable of making small amounts of vitamin K and two of the B-complex vitamins—biotin and pantothenic acid— none of these vitamins are made in adequate amounts. Ultimately, you will need to obtain your vitamins through eating and secondarily through vitamin supplementation. Remember also that each vitamin is not in every food. You need a balanced diet to get them all, and obviously, an excess of one vitamin will in no way compensate for a deficiency of another.

Vitamins are broken down into two categories: fat soluble and water soluble. The former can be stored in the body, but the latter cannot be stored in significant quantities and so must be renewed on a daily basis. The fat-soluble vitamins are A, D, E, and K. The water-soluble vitamins include vitamin C and the eight B-complex vitamins.

Although theoretically a well-balanced diet could provide sufficient quantities of all the vitamins you need, in practice few people eat that well, and even those who do may be able to optimize

---

Fat-soluble vitamins:
    Vitamin A
    Vitamin D
    Vitamin E
    Vitamin K

Water-soluble vitamins:
    Vitamin C
    Thiamin (vitamin B_1)
    Riboflavin (vitamin B_2)
    Niacin (vitamin B_3)
    Pyridoxine (vitamin B_6)
    Biotin
    Pantothenic acid and Pantethine
    Folic acid
    Vitamin B_{12}

their health in certain directions by following a prudent program of vitamin supplementation. This certainly does not mean going in for megadoses of everything in sight, but there is sufficient evidence from thousands of studies to recommend a relatively modest vitamin program that would be supplemental to a first-class diet. If you choose not to eat well, don't expect that supplements alone will be able to reverse the damage that will inevitably result.

Now let's look at the individual vitamins. Remember, as I point out their virtues and their known cancer-fighting capacities, that they never work alone. Not only do they need each other, they also need a myriad of other substances that your body consumes or manufactures. It is by interacting with the other nutrients discussed in this book that a vitamin C or E achieves its full power. Even in so elementary a matter as preventing scurvy, vitamin C alone is not nearly as effective as vitamin C combined with bioflavonoids.

Vitamin A

IMMUNITY BOOSTER AND CANCER FIGHTER

Many decades ago, vitamin A was referred to as the "anti-infective vitamin." A great deal of work since then on its capacity to tune up the immune system shows that that wasn't such a bad name. The current fashion is to call it the immune-factor vitamin. Vitamin A boosts immune responses in the elderly, in patients who have undergone surgery, and in those who have parasitic infections. At least a dozen clinical trials have demonstrated that vitamin A supplementation reduces the likelihood of death among children with severe measles or among those who live where vitamin A deficiency is extremely common.

Vitamin A is essential for vision—particularly night vision. In ancient times, night blindness was treated with the juice from cooked liver, which is, indeed, an outstanding source of vitamin A. Vitamin A's alternative name, retinol, indicates that it is an alcohol involved in the functioning of the retina of the eye.

From the point of view of our interest in cancer, vitamin A has some powerful effects that strongly suggest its importance in stopping malignancies before they start. It is considered to be a prime regulator of cell development. This means it encourages the proper division and healthy growth of cells, leading eventually to cell differentiation, the essential process by which a cell becomes firmly wedded to its duties, whether it be as nerve cell, heart cell, liver cell, or digestive tract cell. Cells that have been given such a lifetime occupation are far less likely to turn malignant.

Vitamin A is extremely important for the health of the skin. It helps stimulate growth of the base level of skin cells both externally and internally. Adequate levels of vitamin A are essential for the health of the mucous membranes of the nose, eyes, bladder, vagina, and intestinal tract.

If Vitamin A is so essential to the structural integrity of these areas, we would expect problems when supplies are low. In fact, low levels apparently permit precancerous changes in skin and mucous membranes to get started. This observation has quite naturally led to research to determine whether the administration of vitamin A can help in reversing such premalignancies.

To date, results from two studies at the M. D. Anderson Cancer Center in Houston, Texas, have answered with a firm yes. By giving patients high doses of a form of vitamin A called 13-*cis*-retinoic acid, or isoretinoin, the researchers were able to reverse cell changes in the mouth that would in all probability have led to cancer. After these reversals, the researchers gave the same people low maintenance doses of 13-*cis*-retinoic acid and succeeded in preventing any further premalignant changes. In effect, the administration of a vitamin was stopping the development of a cancer right in front of the scientists' eyes.

A team of researchers in Milan, Italy, also concluded that clinical studies already done have shown vitamin A as active in "reversing skin and oral precancer, in preventing primary skin cancer, superficial bladder cancer, and second primary tumors associated with head and neck or lung cancers." More than 30 trials of vitamin A compounds are now in progress or are being planned, so it cannot be said that the medical community is ignoring the vitamin corner when it comes to cancer prevention.

SOURCES AND SUPPLEMENTS

Basically, vitamin A comes either as preformed vitamin A, which is mostly found in meats and other animal products, or as provitamin A, which refers to various precursor substances, such as beta carotene, that can be converted to vitamin A once they're inside the body. We've already discussed the carotenoids, including beta carotene, at length in Chapter 6, so in this chapter we're sticking to preformed vitamin A.

As you've just seen, vitamin A is a vigorous and important agent of good health and cancer prevention. It's also one of the vitamins that must be taken with caution, if you decide to ingest it in supplement form. Vitamin A is stored in the body quite readily and is not easily excreted. Some adults take a daily dose of 25,000 international units of it for days or even weeks, and many people do so when they're fighting colds or other infections. Long-term supplementation at such a level might eventually lead to toxicity, however, which can cause fatigue, nausea, vomiting, headache, liver damage, impairment of musclar coordination, and loss of hair. Such symptoms are normally reversible. Pregnant women, however, should

Vitamin A–Rich Foods

Sources	RE*
Apricots, raw, 3 medium	277
Broccoli, boiled, ½ cup	108
Brussels sprouts, boiled, ½ cup	56
Cantaloupe, raw, 1 cup pieces	5,458
Carrots, boiled, ½ cup	1,915
Chard, swiss, boiled, ½ cup	276
Chickory greens, raw, ½ cup chopped	360
Collard greens, boiled, ½ cup	349
Guava, raw, medium	71
Kale, boiled, ½ cup	481
Mango, raw, medium	806
Papaya, raw, medium	612
Pumpkin, canned, ½ cup	2,691
Spinach, boiled, ½ cup	737
Sweet potato, baked with skin, medium	2,488
Tomato, red, raw, medium	77
Turnip greens, boiled, ½ cup	396
Watermelon, raw, 1 cup	58

*RE-retinol equivalent in micrograms.

Pharmacist's Corner

■ It is safe for healthy adults to take a dosage of 10,000 international units of vitamin A daily. Since it is a totally fat soluble vitamin, it is better absorbed if taken with a meal.

■ Vitamin A is needed for morphogenesis, the changes that occur in the cells and tissues of a developing fetus, but scientists are not sure what dosage is safe and what dosage is necessary during pregnancy. For that reason, pregnant women and women of childbearing age should take only 5,000 international units of vitamin A daily. Vitamin A is present in prenatal vitamin–mineral supplements; therefore, no additional supplementation is necessary if you are taking one.

■ Alcohol consumption and both liver and kidney disease can increase vitamin A's toxic potential.

■ Mineral-oil laxatives inhibit the absorption of vitamin A and other fat-soluble vitamins. Patients who are taking mineral-oil laxatives need to consult their physician about supplementation.

probably not supplement with a dosage of vitamin A greater than 5,000 IUs. For the rest of you, my advice is not to supplement for any length of time with more than 10,000 international units of vitamin A daily. Whatever you do, don't be like the Arctic explorer who, having shot a polar bear, sat down and feasted on its liver. He took in a toxic dose of more than 1 million international units of vitamin A and died on the spot.

VITAMIN C

No doubt about it, vitamin C, also known as ascorbic acid, is a heck of a powerful vitamin. There's plenty of evidence that it offers protection against cardiovascular disease, protects us from some of the effects of pollution, prevents gum disease, and helps manufacture collagen, the protein that—through its effects on connective tissue, cartilage, and tendons—literally holds our bodies together. Of course, vitamin C helps prevent cancer.

Although we desperately need vitamin C, it is a vitamin of which the human race all too frequently suffers deficiencies. We cannot store it very efficiently, and we are one of the few animals on this planet that do not manufacture our own supply within ourselves. Every milligram of vitamin C that your body has ever had available for use was metabolized from a food source or a supplement. Since this is an enormously useful vitamin, properly famous as an antioxidant, we should be taking in at least the recommended daily allowance (RDA) every day—and probably somewhat more.

People have always suffered from vitamin C deficiency. In its most extreme form, it is called scurvy, and travelers were congenitally subject to it on long sea voyages. A lack of fresh fruits and vegetables initiated the disease. Scurvy resulted in bleeding gums, muscle wasting, and poor wound healing. If dietary inadequacy continued, the sufferers' teeth would fall out, their bones and muscles would ache, their immune systems would collapse, overmastering fatigue and depression would set in, and eventually death would come, which, by that point, was probably a relief.

In the 1750s, James Lind, a British naval physician, conducted one of the first clinical trials in medical history. He made his experiment on the scurvy-plagued sailors of the British navy. He put limes in the diet of one group of sailors and excluded them from another group's diet. Then on the long sea voyage that followed, he observed the results. The lime consumers remained healthy because of the presence of the unnamed and unknown vitamin C that was contained in the fruit; the unfortunate seamen who were limeless suffered all the agonies of scurvy. After some years of characteristic bureaucratic procrastination, the navy began to ship limes in every ship, and the British sailors, now scurvyless, acquired the nickname of limeys.

ANTIOXIDANT PROTECTOR

You're probably aware that vitamin C is one of the body's main antioxidant protectors. Many free-radical reactions that could initiate cancers and cardiovascular disease are stymied by vitamin C's presence in your tissues and cells. Of course, it works best in conjunction with such other antioxidants as vitamin E, beta carotene, and selenium. One of vitamin C's major activities is restoring vitamin E to full potency after the vitamin gets into bruising entanglements with free radicals.

Scientists have long suspected that vitamin C helps protect against cancer because of population studies that show that people who eat foods high in it lower their risk of various cancers, especially of the stomach and esophagus. The fact that vitamin C can block the formation of nitrosamine, a major carcinogen that is produced in the body when we eat foods containing nitrites (especially bacon and other cured-meat products), is certainly responsible for some part of its cancer-preventive effects.

Cancer researchers in England have also shown that vitamin C has the ability to reduce the rate of cancerous changes in the cells of the stomach caused by stomach juices. The conclusion was that 4 grams (4,000 milligrams) of vitamin C a day could reduce the rate of cancer-promoting change by nearly 50 percent. It probably isn't surprising, therefore, that a recent study of 41,800 postmenopausal women in Iowa found that the women who had higher intakes of vitamin C, vitamin E, and beta carotene had a markedly lower risk of contracting cancer of the mouth, esophagus, and stomach.

Pharmacist's Corner

■ Medical professionals largely agree that taking a vitamin C supplement of 500 milligrams daily is both safe and desirable. At doses higher than that, remember to take vitamin E and selenium as well; there is a complex interplay between the antioxidants.

■ Ester C is a well-absorbed, well-tolerated source of vitamin C that is buffered, preventing any possible vitamin C–related gastrointestinal distress. Many manufacturers provide this enhanced, patented form of Vitamin C in powders, tablets, and capsules.

■ Because they support the activity of each other, purchase a supplement that contains both vitamin C and bioflavinoids.

Vitamin C–Rich Foods

Sources	Milligrams
Avocado, Florida	24
Banana	10
Broccoli, boiled, ½ cup	58
Brussels sprouts, boiled, ½ cup	48
Cabbage, red, cooked, ½ cup	22
Cauliflower, boiled, ½ cup	34
Grapefruit, pink and red, medium	47
Guava, raw, medium	165
Kale, boiled, ½ cup	27
Kiwi, raw, medium	75
Mango, medium	57
Orange, raw, navel, medium	80
Orange juice, fresh, 8 fluid ounces	124
Peas, green, boiled, ½ cup	11
Pineapple, raw, 1 cup pieces	24
Potato, baked with skin	20
Raspberries, raw, 1 cup	31
Snow peas, frozen, 3 ounces	24
Soybeans, green, boiled, ½ cup	15
Spinach, boiled, ½ cup	16
Strawberries, raw, 1 cup	85
Tomato, red, raw	24

In parts of Asia, it has been shown that supplementation with vitamin C can dramatically lower the risk of gastric and esophageal cancer. In these cases, there may be an actual vitamin deficiency. Even in America, though, surveys have shown that one third of the population does not take in the RDA for vitamin C—and that RDA is almost certainly too low to begin with.

Although Linus Pauling's contention that high-dose vitamin C (in the range of 10 grams per day) could actually treat cancer has not been confirmed and seems dubious to many oncologists (including me), the evidence for vitamin C's protective effects seems strong. The studies I've already described barely scratch the surface. Briefly, let's consider the evidence relating to three different types of cancer.

BREAST CANCER

A 1990 analysis of all the various studies on breast cancer found that of all dietary factors, vitamin C had the strongest association with reduced cancer risk.

CERVICAL CANCER

Studies have shown that women with low levels of vitamin C consumption have a fourfold increase of cervical cancer over women with high levels. In addition, women with precancerous changes in their cervix (cervical dysplasia) have significantly lower blood levels of vitamin C than do women with healthy cervixes. There is little or no question that this demonstrates a protective effect for the vitamin.

COLON CANCER

In 1987, the National Cancer Institute, a division of the National Institutes of Health in Bethesda, Maryland, did a study demonstrating that vitamin C inhibited the creation of cancer-causing chemicals by bacteria in the colon. Since high-fiber diets are often rich in vitamin C, this might be a further explanation of the protection fiber has long been observed to provide against cancers of the colon. In any event, I think it's no surprise that six studies have demonstrated a reduction in colon cancer risk with high intake of vitamin C.

ONE LAST WORD

The relation of vitamin C to health and cancer prevention seems significant, but if one more demonstration of that fact is necessary, I will conclude with a statistical analysis conducted by J. E. Enstrom, Ph.D., of the University of California, Los Angeles (UCLA) School of Public Health in 1992. Dr. Enstrom was harvesting the fruits of a national database that had collected extensive diet and nutrition information from 11,348 adults and had then kept track of their health for more than a decade. Deciding to concentrate on vitamin C, the UCLA researcher divided these folks into three groups:

- Individuals who took in less than 50 milligrams daily
- Individuals who took in 50 milligrams or more from food
- Individuals who took in 50 milligrams or more from food, plus regular vitamin C supplementation, usually in the form of pills containing several hundred milligrams

The results were striking. Men in the third group had a total number of deaths 35 percent lower than comparable groups in the total U.S. population. Their cardiovascular mortality was 42 percent lower. And their death rate from cancers of all types was 22 percent lower. Women in the high vitamin C group also had significant benefits: a 10 percent drop in total mortality, a 25 percent decline in heart disease deaths, and a 15 percent reduction in cancer deaths. The large size of the study and the lengthy period of time over which it was conducted make these results particularly significant.

SOURCES AND SUPPLEMENTS

Vitamin C is extremely widely distributed in the plant kingdom, present in virtually all fruits and vegetables. See the box on page 181 for some of the most common sources of C. Supplementation in the range of 500 to 1,000 milligrams a day is also not a bad idea!

VITAMIN E

People have been saying nice things about vitamin E since the 1940s, but only recently has it achieved de facto respectability. Surveys show that four of every five doctors take vitamin E supplements daily, a vote of confidence that isn't easy to ignore. Many scientists now believe that vitamin E is an antioxidant so essential to life that very few members of the animal kingdom—and certainly not you and I—could survive without it.

Vitamin E is particularly important because as a fat-soluble vitamin, it takes its antioxidant power into places that most of the other antioxidants don't go. For instance, vitamin E gets incorporated into the fatty portion of cell membranes. Once there, it delivers an on-site protection service. It also travels around the body guarding the lipid (fat) molecules that circulate in our bloodstream from free-radical damage.

In your fat cells, vitamin E has plenty to defend you against. Heavy metals like mercury, cadmium, and lead are hammering at the door. Toxins, including carbon tetrachloride, benzene, ozone, and nitrous oxide, are invading your cells with their carcinogenic potential—and what about all the other ingredients in cigarette smoke and polluted air? Happily for those of us who manage to maintain high vitamin E levels, it provides the lungs with some protection from oxidative damage caused by smoking and environmental pollution.

Vitamin E also helps maintain the biological activity of vitamin A, protecting it from oxidative destruction, just as E itself is protected by vitamin C. Although for organizational reasons I'm obliged to explain each vitamin separately, the antioxidants inside you work as a team, unable to function effectively without one another.

FRIEND TO THE IMMUNE SYSTEM

Vitamin E is a vigorous stimulator of the immune system. It helps to protect the thymus gland and guards white blood cells from damage. Numerous studies have shown that the immune systems of animals sing when vitamin E levels are high and sour when they're low. In one study, a group of aging mice were given vitamin E at 17 times the level normally present in their diet. Their immune systems' function rose to levels associated with young mice. In another mouse study, infusions of vitamin E enhanced their resistance to bacterial infections appreciably.

Of course, vitamin E's formidable antioxidant punch is, in and of itself, an immunity-enhancing attribute. Recent research has shown that vitamin E can reduce levels of prostaglandin E_2 (PGE-2), the inflammatory prostaglandin that we talked about in Chapters 3 and 7. That's important because PGE-2 tends to damp down immune function. If vitamin E is so powerful, surely it ought to provide some cancer protection? I thought you'd never ask.

UP AGAINST CANCER

The most interesting recent study of cancer and vitamin E was conducted by a team of Finnish researchers and published in the

Journal of the National Cancer Institute in 1997. The Finnish team was interested in prostate cancer, and they followed the fortunes of 29,000 men, some of whom had been randomly assigned to take 75 international units of vitamin E daily. After 8 years, the rate at which prostate cancer had been diagnosed was 32 *percent lower* among the men who were taking the vitamin E supplements. Their overall death rate from prostate cancer was 41 percent lower. The authors concluded that this "suggests that vitamin E has the potential to prevent one of the most common malignant tumors in the North American and European populations"—which seems a fair assessment.

The study results also struck a note of apparent contradiction. It was found that the incidence of latent prostate cancer detected during autopsies was more or less the same among the men taking vitamin E as among the other men. This contradiction is actually no such thing and, in a sense, is not even disappointing. Prostate cancer is a highly unusual malignancy. The prostate gland is a thick, fibrous little object about the size of a chestnut, and changes that occur inside it, within the so-called prostatic capsule, are not all that readily transmitted to the rest of the body. In the majority of men, after a prostatic malignancy reaches a detectable size, it will still take years or even decades for it to break out of the prostatic capsule and endanger a man's life. Even though 40,000 men die yearly from this disease, it is even more common for men to have it and never find out that they do. When men over the age of 80 die of other causes and are autopsied, more than 30 percent of them are found to have had prostate cancer.

Clearly, then, if vitamin E keeps latent prostate cancers below the level of detectability, it is doing nearly as much to lower the mortality rate as it would if it stopped the creation of prostatic cancer cells in the first place.

Here are a few more indications of vitamin E's potential:

- As far back as 1984, researchers observed that vitamin E levels in the blood were lower in men who developed lung and colorectal cancers.
- Various population studies have shown that low intakes of vitamin E and the carotenoids are associated with increased

risk of oral cancer. A recent study, for example, demonstrated that three of our major antioxidants are capable of causing the regression of oral leukoplakia, a premalignant form of oral cancer that's very common among smokers. Over a 6-month period, beta carotene given at 40 milligrams per day, vitamin A given at 100,000 international units per week, or vitamin E given at 80 milligrams per week caused a significant regression of the premalignant lesions. In hamsters as well, an actual regression of oral cancer has been demonstrated using vitamin E.

* A very interesting Finnish study showed that women with the highest levels of vitamin E were only half as likely as women with the lowest levels to develop breast or uterine cancer.

That final study has encouraged me to give vitamin E to patients with breast cancer. Anne Lamont, a patient of mine, is a case in point. When she first came to see me, she was 37 years old, and her sister had died of breast cancer at the age of 43. She herself had a breast lump, which turned out to be a breast condition with no relation to malignancies of the breast—a benign fibroadenoma. I screened Anne to see if she had any mutation in the BRCA—or breast cancer—genes. We found none, thus ruling out that type of genetic tendency to breast cancer, but Anne was still very concerned about the possibility of breast cancer and wanted to know what preventive steps I could suggest.

There was a lot to tell her. Vitamin E was near the top of the list, especially after I checked her blood levels of it and found them to be very low. I also mentioned yet another study, done by R. S. London, which showed that 600 units of vitamin E taken daily improves the ratio of progesterone to estradiol in the blood—a very good thing—for this hormonal alteration would tend to lessen the severity of the type of fibrocystic disease that Anne had.

I told Anne to put a lot of wheat germ, whole grains, leafy vegetables, broccoli, and Brazil nuts in her diet. Since her job as a saleswoman for a major corporation required her to travel frequently, I suggested that she supplement with 400 international units of vitamin E daily.

Anne also took steps to increase her level of selenium, taking 100 micrograms of it daily in supplemental form. She also began taking CoQ_{10} (100 milligrams daily). I encouraged her not to cook with margarine, because of its trans fatty acids; I said that butter would be better, and best of all would be olive oil, the king of cooking oils. Finally, I encouraged Anne to learn how to do meditation and visualizaton on a daily basis (see Chapter 20).

After six months on this program, Anne reported to me that she had never felt better in her life. Soon after, her breast surgeon announced a marked decrease in the extent of fibrocystic breast disease she had. I am convinced that the changes Anne has made in her diet and lifestyle not only will help protect her from breast cancer but will also have favorable effects on her physical and mental well-being that will reverberate through the rest of her life.

SOURCES AND SUPPLEMENTS

It has been estimated that most Americans get about 15 international units of vitamin E in their daily diet, which seems woefully inadequate. The vitamin is simply not that well supplied in the foods we eat. Moreover, some of the foods that do contain marginally satisfactory amounts of E—vegetable oils, seeds, nuts, and grains—are also high in polyunsaturated fatty acids. These fats have been convincingly associated with higher cancer risk, perhaps in part because once they get inside us, polyunsaturates are prone to suffer considerable oxidative damage. In addition, the food-processing techniques that became common in the early years of this century leech much of the vitamin E out of grains and oils, so to speak. These techniques, the basis of the packaged-food empires, continue to degrade our food supply to this day. Try to avoid processed foods. They contain what you don't need and they can do you harm.

Of all the major vitamins, vitamin E is the hardest to obtain purely through a carefully chosen diet. I believe most people would benefit from taking at least 100 international units—but not more than 400 international units—of vitamin E daily in supplemental form.

Pharmacist's Corner

■ Vitamin E is available in both natural and synthetic forms. *dl* before the chemical name would designate a manufactured form (*dl*-alpha tocopherol) and studies have demonstrated that this form of vitamin E is less active in heart muscle and brain tissue. Other studies have demonstrated that a form of vitamin E known as gamma has particularly strong anticancer activity. The gamma form is not found in a typical vitamin E supplement but only in the mixed version. Therefore, a preferred vitamin E supplement would be labeled as vitamin E mixed tocopherols and would include the following: *d*-alpha, *d*-beta, *d*-gamma, and *d*-delta tocopherols.

■ The dosage of vitamin E varies according to its use. To help prevent Alzheimer's disease, clinicians use massive doses of vitamin E. Although vitamin E is nontoxic, the best dosage for stimulating immune function and therefore for cancer prevention seems to range from 200 to 400 international units once a day with food. Vitamin E may slow blood clotting. People who are taking anticoagulants, such as warfarin (Coumadin), should consult a physician before taking vitamin E.

■ As mentioned in Chapter 6, large doses of beta carotene can deplete vitamin E levels in the blood. If your doctor has prescribed a dose of beta carotene in the range of 50,000 international units daily or more you should take a vitamin E supplement as well.

■ Chronic use of mineral-oil laxatives interferes with the absorption of vitamin E, so patients taking these laxatives must discuss vitamin E supplementation with their physician.

VITAMIN D

SKIN, BONES, AND MORE

Vitamin D had never been exactly a glamour vitamin, and most people know little about it. You may have heard that exposure to sunlight can create some of it in your skin. If you're interested in bone preservation—and I know most women are—you will probably have heard that desirable levels of it, combined with sufficient calcium, will help you maintain a healthy skeleton for a lifetime. This vitamin has some additional significance, though.

In the 1990s, there has been some movement toward regarding vitamin D as a cancer preventive vitamin. One of the earliest, and still most intriguing, observations was that those areas of the United States with the highest breast and colon cancer mortality rates were also the areas with the least amount of natural sunlight. Since vitamin D is present in relatively few foods, most of us obtain a high percentage of our total intake from this vitamin's remarkable capacity to be synthesized in our skin from the ultraviolet (UV) rays of the sun. There is now a scientific consensus that very little of it gets absorbed this way during the winter months in northern climates—the days are too short and the sun is too shrouded.

Moreover, we now know that vitamin D deficiency is extremely common. A study done at the Massachusetts General Hospital in Boston detected vitamin D deficiency in 57 percent of 290 consecutive patients who were admitted to the hospital. Even among those who showed no known risk factors for such a deficiency, it was found that 42 percent were vitamin D deficient.

How do we solve the vitamin D problem? Obviously, a certain amount of fresh air and sunshine is good for people. Even if people could be persuaded to change their lifestyle, however, I wouldn't go around encouraging them to get as much sunshine as possible. The threat of skin cancer is very real. Vitamin D is a nutrient that needs to be obtained by food and supplement.

Here is a brief sampling of the work—still very preliminary—being done to determine whether vitamin D really does have a relation to the prevention of cancer:

- **Prostate cancer:** A recent study found that men with elevated risk of prostate cancer had lower summer levels of 1,25-dihyroxyvitamin-D (the active form of vitamin D).
- **Colon cancer:** The famous Harvard Nurses' Study, which follows the fortunes of 89,000 female nurses, has shown a significant association between total intake of vitamin D and lower risk of colorectal cancer.

The Harvard study seems to provide some confirmation

of the work done by researchers at the University of California at San Diego. They analyzed the data on 2,000 men who were subjects in a Western Electric Health Study done at the company's Chicago facility in 1957. In this study, detailed dietary histories were taken a number of times, and the men's physical condition was carefully monitored for 19 years. When the men in this study who eventually suffered colorectal cancer were analyzed, they were found to differ in only two respects from their fellow workers: their dietary intake of calcium and vitamin D had been much lower. Statistical analysis then showed that the men with the lowest dietary intake of calcium and vitamin D had 2.7 times the risk of colorectal cancer of those with the highest intake.

Yet another study conducted over 8 years found that high blood levels of vitamin D correlated with a lowered risk for colon cancer. Dutch scientists have also speculated that vitamin D may inhibit cell proliferation in the colorectal area.

The above research is beginning to look impressive, especially the colon cancer studies. Lab work has shown that the active form of vitamin D will inhibit the multiplication of cells from human colon cancer metastases in the test tube.

SOURCES AND SUPPLEMENTS

Vitamin D is the only vitamin for which we depend to a major extent on something other than food (that is, sunlight) for our supply. It is fairly sparsely represented in the food supply, the main sources being fatty fish, egg yolks, and liver. Because milk is fortified with vitamin D, milk and dairy products are good sources. There has been speculation that the reason why the Japanese do not have high levels of colon cancer in spite of their northern latitude and consequent paucity of sunlight is that they more than make up the difference through high consumption of cold-water fatty fish.

Supplementation with vitamin D must be done carefully. Inappropriately high dosing can have extremely toxic effects with such symptoms as nausea, headache, and fatigue, quite secondary to the possibility of liver and kidney damage and even death. The RDA

Pharmacist's Corner

■ Vitamin D is a safe and healthy supplement at 400 international units daily. Take it with food, because it is fat soluble. Studies indicate that postmenopausal women with osteoporosis may need to take 600 to 800 international units of vitamin D daily for optimal calcium use.

■ **Drug interaction:** Steroidal anti-inflammatory drugs, such as Prednisone and Decadron, can cause vitamin D depletion. Drugs used to absorb cholesterol, such as Questran, can absorb and deplete vitamin D and other fat-soluble vitamins (A, E, and K.) Mineral-oil laxatives can also deplete D.

for vitamin D is 400 international units. Several studies have shown that supplementation up to 1,000 international units daily is safe. I would definitely not go higher.

THE B VITAMINS

The B vitamins are a study in themselves, so I am not going to discuss them one by one. Instead, we'll simply take a brief look at some of the cancer-proven qualities that scientists have noticed in vitamin B_{12} and in folic acid, part of the B vitamin family. Of course, you shouldn't take this restrictive approach on our part as an excuse to think that the other B vitamins aren't important. This whole vitamin grouping isn't called the B complex for nothing. You need all the B vitamins in your diet, and you should be aware that they often work together.

The vitamin B_{12} story can be summarized quickly. One single study's results have impressively associated it with folic acid in offering protection to smokers. Researchers had noticed before that smokers generally had abnormally low levels of both these vitamins. In this study, 73 men who had put in 20 or more pack-years of smoking were found to have potentially precancerous changes in their bronchial tissues. (A pack-year is 1 year smoking one pack a day; 1 year smoking 2 packs a day would be two pack-years, and so on.) The men were divided into two groups, one receiving 500 micrograms of B_{12} and 10 milligrams of folic acid daily and the other receiving a placebo. After 4 months, the men taking those two B vitamins showed a marked reduction in the number of cells in their bronchial passages that were precancerous—a potentially lifesaving physical change.

Meanwhile, studies of folic acid alone suggest that it is probably protective against a wide variety of cancers. Low levels have been associated with increased risk for cancer of the cervix, colon, rectum, lung, esophagus, and brain. Folic acid is necessary for deoxyribonucleic acid (DNA) repair and also for vigorous immune function.

Interest in folic acid's relation to colon cancer has been particularly intense. For example, a large study done on 9,940 men and 15,984 women showed that those who consumed the highest levels of folic acid in their food were 29 to 35 percent less likely to develop premalignant adenomas of the colon. The same study reported that drinking as little as two alcoholic drinks per day increased the risk of such premalignancies by 85 percent. These two apparently distinct statistical associations are in all probability closely related. Alcohol is well known for destroying folic acid in the body.

One other extremely interesting study should be mentioned. This was a group of women who had cervical dysplasia, the abnormal cellular changes of the cervix that result in a positive Pap (Papanicolaou) smear and indicate a sharply increased risk of cancer. Researchers gave the women 10 milligrams of folic acid a day for 2 months, which, in that time period, eliminated most of the precancerous cells that they had discovered initially.

I believe folic acid is powerful medicine, and the American medical establishment is coming around to that view, too, partly because supplementation with folic acid has been shown to decrease birth defects! Supplementation with 400 micrograms of folic acid daily is very reasonable for just about anyone. Pregnant women might consider doubling that dose.

Folic Acid–Rich Foods

Source	Micrograms
Artichoke, boiled, medium	61
Asparagus, boiled, 1/2 cup (6 spears)	132
Avocado, Florida, medium	162
Brewer's yeast, 1 tablespoon	315
Brussels sprouts, boiled, 1/2 cup	47
Chicken liver, simmered, 3.5 ounces	770
Chickpeas, boiled, 1 cup	282
Collard greens, frozen, 1/2 cup	65
Lentils, cooked, 1 cup	358
Lima beans, boiled, 1 cup	156
Peas, green, boiled, 1/2 cup	57
Pinto beans, boiled, 1 cup	294
Romaine lettuce, raw, 1 cup shredded	76
Soybean flour, low fat, 1 cup	361
Soy nuts, dry roasted, 1/2 cup	176
Spinach, boiled, 1/2 cup	85
Turnip greens, boiled, 1/2 cup	85

A COMPLETE VITAMIN PROGRAM

I think two things are pretty obvious. First, there is an intimate, inverse relationship between risk for cancer and intake of vitamins. If you take many vitamins, you will have less cancer. Second, fruits and vegetables are the foods that have the highest endowment of these vitamins. These are not really surprising conclusions, but even if you've heard the vitamin story a hundred times before, that doesn't make the message any less true.

I'm fairly confident that by the time you finish this book, you'll be eating more fruits and vegetables than you were before you started it. As for supplementation, I recommend it, as long as it's done in a prudent manner. We don't have the information yet that would justify megadoses of vitamins and minerals. We do have very solid evidence demonstrating that daily multivitamins and modest

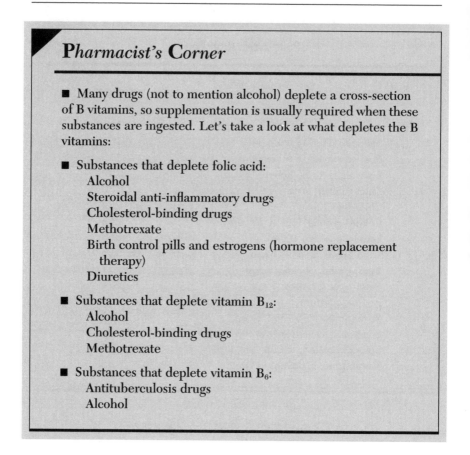

Pharmacist's Corner

■ Many drugs (not to mention alcohol) deplete a cross-section of B vitamins, so supplementation is usually required when these substances are ingested. Let's take a look at what depletes the B vitamins:

■ Substances that deplete folic acid:
  Alcohol
  Steroidal anti-inflammatory drugs
  Cholesterol-binding drugs
  Methotrexate
  Birth control pills and estrogens (hormone replacement therapy)
  Diuretics

■ Substances that deplete vitamin B_{12}:
  Alcohol
  Cholesterol-binding drugs
  Methotrexate

■ Substances that deplete vitamin B_6:
  Antituberculosis drugs
  Alcohol

additional amounts of some of the major vitamins and minerals are protective against most major illnesses, including cancer. A typical multivitamin formulation that we stand behind is in the box on page 195. I would be lacking in candor if I didn't tell you that when I talk to doctors, 9 times out of 10, they tell me they're taking supplements. If you are not eating at least six to eight servings of fruits and vegetables daily, most likely you should take supplements, too.

Preferred Multivitamin Formula (Including Minerals)

Vitamin or Mineral	Amount
Vitamin A	5,000 international units
Vitamin D	400 international units
Vitamin C	500 milligrams
Vitamin B_1	100 milligrams
Vitamin B_2	50 milligrams
Vitamin B_6	25 milligrams
Vitamin B_{12}	500 micrograms
Niacin	10 milligrams
Niacinamide	150 milligrams
Pantothenic acid	500 milligrams
Folic acid	400 micrograms
Biotin	300 micrograms
Choline	100 milligrams
Inositol	100 milligrams
Para-amino benzoic acid (PABA)	50 milligrams
Vitamin E (mixed natural)	200 international units
Calcium	500 milligrams
Magnesium	500 milligrams
Potassium	99 milligrams
Iodine	150 micrograms
Manganese (aspartate)	10 milligrams
Copper (gluconate)	2 milligrams
Boron (chelate)	1 milligram
Zinc	20 milligrams
Molybdenum (chelate)	100 micrograms
Chromium	200 micrograms
Selenium	200 micrograms
Vanadium (chelate)	25 micrograms
Bioflavonoids	100 milligrams

CHAPTER 16

MINERALS

*The longer I live the less confidence
I have in drugs and the greater is my
confidence in the regulation and
administration of diet and regimen.*

—JOHN REDMAN COXE

Without minerals, the human organism is entirely inconceivable. A little bit of this or that rock is one of your natural building blocks, a traveler circulating from cell to cell down the pathways of your veins, perhaps the provoker of some crucial enzymatic reaction. That being so, it's sensible to take shortages and excesses of important minerals quite seriously. Would it surprise you to learn that such imbalances can critically affect the functioning of your body—perhaps even the continuance of your life?

I know that many people imagine that minerals are second-class citizens in the body, obscure little metabolic workers far below vitamins in the hierarchy of everything—but they aren't at all. What would you use for a skeleton without calcium? What would happen to your immune functions without zinc?

The list of can't-live-without-them minerals is indeed a long one. For us, however, it will be more than sufficient to look into what little is known about the relationship of minerals to cancer. I say that little is known, but there are certainly at least three minerals worth describing at some length because of the clearly protective role they have against certain cancers. Before we describe them, let's set the stage with a brief sketch of the mineral playing field.

THE MINERAL BACKGROUND

There are two categories of minerals. The first are called macronutrients because they're needed in such large amounts by the body, and they include calcium, phosphorus, magnesium, sodium, potassium, sulfur, and chloride. The second category is trace minerals, many of which are extremely important even though the body requires them in only minute quantities. They include selenium, zinc, iron, copper, manganese, iodine, chromium, molybdenum, boron, vanadium, and silicon.

Mineral deficiencies are definitely more common in our diet than are vitamin deficiencies. Pregnant and nursing women have a greater need for certain minerals and can easily run short. Elderly people have difficulty absorbing some minerals. Commonly prescribed drugs, such as loop diuretics and thiazide diuretics, can cause mineral losses and produce mineral imbalances.

Rather intriguingly, the part of the world you live in can radically affect your likelihood of having a proper supply of certain critical minerals. This is because the mineral levels in the food you eat will be affected by the mineral levels in the soil, and those levels are far from uniform. If there are deficiencies, they will show up in both the local crops and farm animals. Some countries in the Middle East, such as Iran, for example, are deficient in zinc. Selenium, a particularly important trace mineral, is found in deficient levels in the soil of New Zealand, Finland, Serbia, and sizable areas of China and the United States.

We will shortly see that such deficiencies produce far from trivial results, but let's look now at the first of our three cancer preventive minerals.

CALCIUM

THE BODY IN GENERAL

You remember that mother told you to drink your milk. Although we now know that milk has disadvantages for many people, mother's dietary prescription was far from a bad idea. After all, milk is a pretty good calcium delivery system, and calcium is essential for human life. Not only is it a major constituent of human bone, it is also needed for a proper heart rate, a healthy skin, muscle contraction, nerve conduction, energy production, blood coagulation, and proper immune function. Calcium is critical in so many areas of the body that at the slightest sign of shortage, your metabolism will draw it out of your skeleton—at whatever cost in weakened bone—and will put that calcium where it's needed most.

How to Get Your Calcium

From food, the richest natural sources are milk, cheese, yogurt, and other dairy products. Other sources include cruciferous and green leafy vegetables, sardines, salmon, and tofu. A variety of calcium supplements exist. Calcium carbonate derived from oyster shell, however, is poorly absorbed, but it may be the best form of calcium for preventing colon cancer because a large portion of it remains in your digestive tract. Calcium carbonate can also be dangerous since lead contamination often occurs. Never supplement with dolomite. Calcium citrate, calcium aspartate, and amino acid chelated calcium are the best forms of calcium supplements, as far as absorption and the prevention of osteoporosis are concerned. Men who eat a good diet probably do not need to take calcium supplementally; for postmenopausal women we recommend 1,500–2,000 milligrams of calcium per day.

See the table below for daily calcium needs from diet and/or supplementation.

Daily Calcium Needs* by Category	Milligrams
From birth to 6 months old	400
6 months to 1 year old	600
1–5 years old	800
6–10 years old	800–1,200
11–23 years old	1,200–1,500
Women, 25–50 years old	1,000
Women, pregnant or lactating	1,200
Women postmenopausal and receiving ERT†	1,000
Women, postmenopausal but not receiving ERT	1,500
Men 25–65 years old	1,000
All men and women over 65 years old	1,500

*Adapted from the National Institutes of Health, Bethesda, Maryland.
†ERT-estrogen replacement therapy.

An awful lot of us have a calcium deficiency, and there are many ways to become deficient. A diet poor in vegetables and dairy products will certainly contribute. Excessive drinking of cola beverages can deplete calcium, and I recommend you drink as little as possible. Bottled water, seltzer water, and iced green tea are good beverage substitutes. Colas are loaded with phosphorus; in excess, this mineral will bind with calcium and make it unavailable for ab-

Calcium-Rich Foods

Food	Serving Size	Calcium Content (milligrams)
Dairy products		
Milk, skim	8 ounces	302
Soy milk plus	8 ounces	500
Yogurt, low fat	8 ounces	415
Cheese		
Mozzarella, part skim	1 ounce	207
Ricotta, part skim	4 ounces	335
Cottage, low fat	4 ounces	78
Fish and shellfish		
Sardines, including bones (canned)	3 ounces	175
Salmon, including bones, pink, (canned)	3 ounces	167
Shrimp, drained (canned)	3 ounces	98
Vegetables		
Broccoli, fresh	1 cup	74
Broccoli, frozen	1 cup	100
Soybeans, fresh	1 cup	131
Turnips, fresh, leaves and stems	1 cup	252
Tofu	4 ounces	106

sorption. Intense exercise without a corresponding increase in calcium intake can cause a deficiency. Postmenopausal women suffer grievously from calcium deficiency, often leading to bone loss, and though this is not the place to discuss the complicated question of bone loss in women, there is little doubt that higher estrogen levels in premenopausal women help prevent calcium excretion. People with kidney and liver disease may have trouble keeping up their calcium levels. The potent diuretic Lasix, used to treat high blood pressure and congestive heart failure, will cause a loss of calcium.

Vitamin D is needed for proper calcium absorption, and many people are deficient in vitamin D, especially the elderly, who eat less food and absorb the nutrients within their food less efficiently. In addition, people who take prescription corticosteroids—drugs prescribed commonly for inflammation, asthma, and such autoimmune disorders as rheumatoid arthritis—may deplete their vitamin D. Finally, African Americans especially and people who are fairly dark skinned do not in general create vitamin D from sunlight as effectively as fairer-skinned people and, if they live in northern latitudes, may easily not absorb enough vitamin D in winter to keep their calcium levels up. Thus, many people may need vitamin D supplements as an aid in absorbing calcium. A reasonable dose is 400 international units daily with food.

YOUR COLON

Studies indicate that calcium helps prevent people at high risk for colon cancer from developing it. Considering the rate of colon cancer in America, we are all at least at an elevated risk. One study of patients with adenomatous colon polyps (a potentially precancerous condition) found that after removal of the polyps, the likelihood of a recurrence decreased radically if the patients received calcium supplements. Those who didn't get calcium saw their polyps return 55 percent of the time, but those who did have a recurrence rate of only 12.9 percent. This was an astonishing difference.

It appears that the colon–calcium connection is mostly a bile acid story. Bile acids, created in the liver from cholesterol, are released from the gallbladder into the small intestine, when we eat fatty foods, to help in the breakdown and absorption of the fatty acids. Unfortunately, large amounts of bile acid put us at risk for colon cancer in at least two different ways. First, there is the bile acid itself, which, with a chemical structure very similar to the cancer-causing polycyclic aromatic hydrocarbons, has measurable carcinogenic effects.

Second, there is a compound called glucuronide that gets bound up and taken along by the bile acid. Glucuronide is an important detoxifier that joins itself in the liver to various substances—drugs, hormones, pesticides, xenobiotics, and so on—that need to be excreted in the urine or feces. Bound to bile acid, glucuronide heads toward the place of elimination together with its toxic cargo. Unfortunately, things can happen before it gets there. Unfriendly bacteria in the colon create an enzyme called B-glucuroni-

◤ Pharmacist's Corner

■ Calcium can decrease the effectiveness of a number of antibiotics. If you are prescribed an antibiotic check with your pharmacist to see if the drug interacts with calcium.

■ Some diuretics, such as furosemide (Lasix), can deplete the body of calcium and other minerals; check with your doctor if you are taking a diuretic to see if you need a calcium or mineral supplement.

■ Steroidal anti-inflammatory drugs interfere with calcium metabolism because of their effects on vitamin D.

■ Eating excessive amounts of protein; drinking diet colas, which are high in phosphorus; and performing constant strenuous exercise can deplete your body of calcium and will increase your dietary need for it.

■ Studies demonstrating calcium's ability to protect against cancer have been performed using calcium carbonate. Calcium carbonate is poorly absorbed, compared with other calcium mineral salts, and it may be the best calcium to take for colon cancer prevention because large amounts of it remain in the intestines. Because calcium citrate, calcium aspartate, and chelated calcium have superior absorptive abilities, however, they are the forms of choice for the prevention of osteoporosis.

See the box on page 201 (How to Get Your Calcium) for suggested dosages.

dase that can detach the carcinogens and toxins from the glucuronide freight train and put them more or less freely in contact with the walls of the colon. The longer the mass of the feces stays in the colon—and if you eat a lot of meat, it will stay a long time—the greater the cancer-forming effect on the colon walls. This high concentration of bile acids and enzymes is typically found in people with precancerous adenomatous polyps, as well as in those with full-blown colon cancer. It is thought that calcium binds up the toxic bile acids released from the liver and reduces their reaction with the colon while holding glucuronide and its unappetizing collection of toxins together in the package. Result: minimal transference to the colon wall.

A number of medical studies offer confirmation of calcium's protective effects. One study of 193 people who had precancerous polyps removed from their colons found that when they were given 1 to 2 grams of calcium daily for 6 months, the distribution of new cells in their colon tissue was normal—unlike a similar group who were given a placebo that had no calcium in it and soon began to re-form precancerous polyps. More than one study has shown that patients who received calcium after colon cancer surgery have an increased survival time. Finally, a study in which patients had had their colon polyps surgically removed investigated the effects of giving these patients wheat-bran fiber and calcium carbonate at a dosage of 250 to 1,500 milligrams of elemental calcium per day after surgery. The results showed significant reductions in fecal bile acid concentrations in the patients who followed this regimen, a very promising response.

Almost 50,000 people die yearly from colon cancer, and I think that some diligent attention to getting enough calcium either by dietary means or by supplementation would cut into that gruesome total quite impressively.

In Japan, where stomach cancer is the major form of cancer, they've found that calcium can help lower the rate. The reason is as follows. The Japanese have a very high salt diet. This causes cell proliferation in the stomach and greatly increases the risk of cancer there. It turns out that calcium (which the Japanese diet somewhat lacks) opposes the action of salt and decreases cell growth in the stomach, with less resulting cancer.

ZINC

Zinc is a trace mineral of enormous significance. The body needs it to produce ribonucleic acid (RNA), deoxyribonucleic acid (DNA), and insulin and to carry out a multitude of life-sustaining enzyme functions. It is primarily obtained from fish and eggs, meat and poultry, beans, mushrooms, yeast, whole grains, seeds, and some nuts. Your body needs about 15 milligrams of zinc daily, but it is safe and often desirable to take higher-potency supplements, up to about 30 milligrams a day. Since zinc is poorly stored in the body, a daily supply from food or supplements is required.

Zinc is needed for wound healing, proper immune function, the formation of bones in young people, blood sugar control, normal functioning of the male sex organs, and an adequate sense of taste

---

Getting Your Zinc

Our ability to absorb zinc decreases with age. This makes it hard for older people to be sure that they are getting enough of the mineral even if they eat a healthy diet. Moreover, zinc is one nutrient that is much more bioavailable in seafood and animal meats than in vegetable sources. Many people following a cancer preventive diet will have decided to limit their consumption of animal foods; in so doing, they may be shortchanging themselves in regard to zinc. In all probability, therefore, supplementation in the neighborhood of 15–30 milligrams a day is a wise measure.

Pharmacist's Corner

■ Calcium and many other minerals can interfere with zinc absorption. As a result, I believe that zinc supplements should be taken alone. Unfortunately, some vitamin manufacturers market a mixture of calcium, magnesium, and zinc. Because of the calcium–zinc interaction, I doubt that much zinc from this combination is absorbed.

■ The phytates in rice, soy and other beans can attach to zinc and decrease its absorption. Never take zinc supplements with these foods.

■ Zinc aspartate, chelated zinc, zinc citrate, and zinc picolinate are well-absorbed forms of the mineral and should be your choice for zinc supplementation.

■ A zinc dosage of 15 milligrams to 30 milligrams once a day is more than adequate.

and smell. Zinc is required for the formation of an important antioxidant called superoxide dismutase. It is also needed if the white blood cells called T-cells—critical cancer killers—are to mature properly. Zinc is famously involved in the immune system. A whole host of enzymes needed for the formation and maturation of immune cells depend on this mineral for their effective functioning.

Perhaps this is why, in a number of studies measuring zinc levels in patients with cancer, low zinc levels were associated with poor immune function and a reduced ability to fight cancer. For example, in a study of 30 patients with cancer of the upper aerodigestive tract, 55 percent had mild zinc deficiency. Associated with that deficiency in these patients was a lower level of natural killer cells. A pattern of deficient zinc has also been found for a number of cancers, including prostate, esophageal and bronchogenic cancer. As we're mentioned, zinc levels were found to be a great deal lower in men with cancer of the prostate than in men with normal prostates. In a study of patients with kidney cancer, zinc levels were also found to be lower than in a sampling of the normal population.

There also appears to be an inverse relationship between levels of zinc and copper in some cancer patients. It is recognized that in the general population, as zinc levels fall, copper levels rise. In one cancer study, it was found that patients with digestive tract cancer had far higher copper levels and far lower zinc levels than did people with benign digestive tract disease or in normal health. So strong was the relationship that the scientists conducting the study suggested that a high serum copper level and a low serum zinc level should be regarded as an additional reliable factor to be weighed in evaluating whether there is a cancer of the digestive tract.

I think that zinc's significance in cancer prevention will be noted more and more. Certainly, its significance in cancer treatment has received due recognition. At the 1995 meeting of the American Society of Clinical Oncologists, it was noted not only that zinc deficiency is common among patients with cancer but that this nutritional lack makes it harder for them to fight the cancer, to heal from medical treatment, and to resist infections that may result from cancer treatments that suppress the immune system. The conclusion: zinc levels should be checked routinely in patients with cancer and addressed in treatment.

SELENIUM

One of the strongest cancer preventing nutrients known is the mineral selenium. Although it is a trace mineral required in the body at the level of only a few hundred micrograms a day, selenium, maintained in the body at an ideal level, is very big stuff: it is one of the most potent antioxidants known, a proven immunostimulant, a component of detoxification, and a powerful protector of the cardiovascular system. In fact, parts of Georgia and the Carolinas afflicted with extremely low selenium soil content have been dubbed the stroke belt of the United States.

The cancer correlation is even more stunning. Researchers tracked down the selenium content of soil from many states of the union. Variations were extremely wide. The lowest levels were in Ohio, and the highest levels were in South Dakota. When they looked up cancer mortality rates for the nation, it turned out that Ohio had a cancer death rate nearly double that of South Dakota.

The same phenomenon has been reported in other nations; the lower the selenium intake, the higher the cancer levels. Some scientists speculating on the ever-fascinating question of low breast cancer levels in the women of Japan have pointed to that island nation's high levels of selenium. A study out of China also reported that people living in low-selenium areas had an increased chance of suffering cancer of the stomach, esophagus, or liver, whereas those in high-selenium areas had a decreased risk.

In fact, selenium got its first shot at fame as an actual cancer preventive because of studies, as noted above, that were conducted in China, a nation that, like the United States, has sizable regions with soil characterized by extreme selenium depletion. One of those regions, Linxian, has some of the highest rates of stomach and esophageal cancer mortality found anywhere in the world. It seemed the perfect setting for a test of nutritional effectiveness in the prevention of cancer. Thirty thousand Chinese were given various combinations of nutrients. After 5.25 years of supplementation, those research subjects who had received beta carotene, vitamin E, and selenium were found to have lower total mortality as well as significant reductions in the incidence of stomach and esophageal cancer.

How Much Selenium?

Selenium is found in meat, particularly such organ meat as liver; however, since the liver is the main organ of detoxification, you should purchase only organic liver, which has little or no pesticide residue in it. Selenium is also in shellfish, saltwater fish, grains (if the soil isn't depleted), garlic and onions, broccoli, seaweed, yeast, eggs, and Brazil nuts.

A safe supplemental dose of selenium—the mineral can cause serious side effects if taken in inappropriately toxic high doses—is 100–200 micrograms for an adult. Some people take it in doses as high as 400–600 micrograms with no reported ill effects, but there is probably no need to supplement selenium at such levels. Everything scientists know so far indicates the mineral will achieve its full cancer preventing potential at 200 micrograms.

Selenium Sources

Nuts*:
Brazil nuts
Cashews

Fish:
Haddock
Lobster
Mackerel
Red snapper
Swordfish
Tuna

Vegetables and Fruits:
Broccoli
Coconut
Garlic
Mushrooms
Soybeans
Sunflower seeds

Dairy products:
Eggs

Meat:
Beef
Turkey
Veal

*Oils, nuts, and seeds can deteriorate. It's best if you refrigerate them.

In yet another Chinese study, people in townships with high rates of liver cancer were given 200 micrograms of selenium daily, whereas a control group of similar high-risk Chinese were not. After only two years, it was found that the incidence of liver cancer had been significantly reduced in the group taking selenium.

Studies on the relationship between selenium intake and cancer incidence continue to pour in. By now, the findings are so startling that this trace mineral, which is taken as a supplement in micrograms, or thousandths of a gram, really ought to be recognized as one of the most essential components of any serious cancer prevention program.

In 1996, an especially interesting study on selenium was published in the *Journal of the American Medical Association.* The study had been designed seven years earlier to determine the relationship between selenium intake and the treatment of two types of skin cancer: basal-cell carcinoma and squamous-cell carcinoma. More than 1,000 people with those conditions were given either 200 micrograms of selenium or a placebo each day. When the researchers uncovered the results, however, they found not what they were looking for but something far more astounding. The mineral had little or no impact on the rate at which new basal- or squamous-cell carcinomas were formed, yet the fortunate group of patients who had been given selenium had a reduced *overall* cancer incidence by a whopping 41 percent and a reduced cancer death rate by 52 percent. The rate of prostate cancer was reduced by 70 percent and the rate of colon cancer stages A, B, and C was reduced by 63 percent. The relatively large size of the study and the deeply significant cuts in death and incidence rates makes it very likely that this piece of work will be one of a number of classic studies in the 1990s that permanently alter the conventional wisdom of medicine.

Selenium's already extensive reputation as a cancer preventive mineral seems well deserved. Together with calcium and zinc, selenium offers you a mineral approach to a cancer-free life that you would probably be foolish to ignore.

CHAPTER 17

GARLIC AND ITS RELATIVES

. . . the weight of evidence is making it look like garlic really is protective against cancer.

—WILLIAM BLOT, PH.D., biostatistician at National Cancer Institute; a division of the National Institutes of Health, Bethesda, Maryland

Garlic—potent medicine in a clove—is both ancient folk wisdom revived and burgeoning modern miracle. When the Egyptian pyramids were being built, workers got a clove of garlic daily for strength, and hundreds of years later, Roman soldiers carried it with them as they marched to the borders of the empire. During World War I, battlefield physicians learned that garlic poultices could help prevent wound infection and used them accordingly. They were only following up Louis Pasteur's discovery in 1858 that garlic could kill bacteria in lab cell cultures. Across the world, garlic has long been a centerpiece of vigorous national cuisines.

Today, garlic and its relatives—onions, scallions, and leeks—are heavily researched. Much good science supports their cardiovascular benefits, and a range of highly intriguing studies devoted to their cancer preventive qualities is giving this food family ever-enhanced cachet. I would suggest, on the basis of present evidence, that along with soy products, cruciferous vegetables, and green tea, the garlic family is among the healthiest of foods and the most promising of anticancer phytonutrients.

Garlic, like its relatives, is a member of the allium family of plants. They are all extremely healthy foods, but most researchers have concluded that garlic contains the highest concentration of the most beneficial allium components. It is thought that more than 100 different compounds in garlic are involved in its effects, but the super constituents appear to be its thiolallyl sulfur-containing compounds, which have tongue-twisting names such as S-allyl cysteine, S-allyl mercaptocysteine, and diallyl sulfide. Commercially aged garlic extract appears to have even more of these sulfur compounds than does garlic that comes in nature's original packaging as garlic cloves, but as numerous scientific investigations have shown, eating the garlic family as food is certainly still strong medicine.

THE HEALTHY STOMACH SAGA

In the 1980s, researchers in Italy wanted to know why the residents of Cagliari, the capital of Sardinia, had so little stomach cancer— about one third as much—compared with their compatriots in northern Italy. They gathered dietary data for three years and found that among Cagliarians, garlic was more frequently eaten than any other single food. The northern Italians of Tuscany and Emilia-Romagna ate garlic once a week, but the folks from Cagliari downed it on average 7.2 times a week. An article in *Hippocrates,* a glossy magazine for doctors that often turns up in their office waiting rooms, reported that University of Cagliari epidemiologist Pierluigi Cocco remarked: "It wouldn't surprise me if they sold more mouthwash here [in Cagliari] than anywhere else in the world."

The association between garlic and cancer protection might not have attracted so much attention if similar news hadn't come out of China in 1987. A study in China's Shandong Province looked at the health effects of garlic, scallions, chives, and onions. Compared to those who ate them rarely, the bigger consumers among the Shandong Chinese showed a 40 percent reduction in the rate of stomach cancer.

It was beginning to seem like a pattern. The hypothesis researchers came up with was that one or more of the allyl sulfide compounds in garlic neutralizes bacterial growth in the stomach. This could be important because it may limit the conversion of foods into nitrosamines, famously potent and widespread carcinogens that require bacterial activity in the intestines for their creation out of the nitrites found in foods. In the opinion of Robert Lin, Ph.D., a noted garlic researcher, sulfhydryl, diallyl sulfides, and polysulfides all have the ability to block this important and deadly conversion.

Actual experimental work was done by University of Texas cancer researchers at the M.D. Anderson Cancer Center in Houston. They tested diallyl sulfide, one of the principal garlic sulfur compounds, on rats. The rats were pretreated with the garlic compound and then fed a substance that usually causes stomach cancer. The experiment demonstrated that diallyl sulfide suppresses two of the specific cell abnormalities that would normally have been produced. Moreover, the higher the dose of the garlic extract the rats were given, the fewer cancerous cell changes occurred. In their report, the M.D. Anderson scientists concluded that diallyl sulfide has pluripotent effects on cancer cells—that is, it works in more ways than one.

CANCER ENEMY

Is garlic merely a stomach cancer preventative? You'll see that this is hardly the case. John Pinto, Ph.D., of the Memorial Sloan-Kettering Cancer Center in New York wrote that "there is growing evidence that garlic or its derivatives may be able to prevent the development of at least six different cancers." He was referring to malignancies of the breast, colon, skin, stomach, esophagus, and prostate.

Dr. Pinto has concentrated on the effects of aged garlic extract on the prostate. He and his team worked with prostate cancer cells that they had exposed to the male hormone testosterone, which is suspected of stimulating the growth of prostatic cancer cells. When the cells were simultaneously exposed to S-allyl mercaptocysteine, a sulfur compound that forms as garlic ages, they broke down and eliminated the testosterone two to four times more rapidly, and they did this without converting it to an even more potent growth-promoting form of testosterone, namely, dihydrotestosterone. Pinto was quoted in 1997 in *Science News* as saying the garlic derivative was "doing the same thing that testosterone deprivation would do." This might promise great improvements in prostate cancer therapy, since there are a number of disadvantages, including temporary impotence, related to the testosterone deprivation therapies that are commonly used to treat prostate cancer.

The medical world is skeptical about isolated studies, but in fact, the reports on the cancer preventive effects of the allium family of vegetables are more in the nature of a flood than a trickle. A 1997 review of the literature found 20 epidemiologic studies investigating the relation of garlic and onion consumption with cancer risk. All the studies except one revealed a statistically significant protective effect.

One rather large research project of this type came from the University of Minnesota School of Public Health. A survey conducted there of the eating habits of 41,000 women found that not only was there a relationship between eating lots of fruits and vegetables and having lowered risk of colon cancer but that there was an especially strong correlation between consumption of garlic and that lowering of risk.

Let's glance at a few of the pearls about garlic and cancer that researchers have thrown down before us:

- In widely reported experiments in the 1990s, Dr. John Milner of Pennsylvania State University was actually able to prevent the development of breast cancer tumors in rats exposed to carcinogens. Among the rats receiving aged garlic extract, only 35 percent developed tumors, whereas in those receiving none, tumor incidence was 90 percent—an astounding difference. Milner also believes that major components of aged garlic extract, such as S-allyl cysteine, can help inhibit lung cancer development in rats.

- Following up on the breast cancer question, G. Li, Ph.D., reported in a 1995 study in *Oncology Reports* on test-tube experiments. He demonstrated that the major sulfur compounds in garlic extract inhibited the growth of precancerous human breast cells and increased levels of glutathione-S-transferase in noncancerous cells. Glutathione-S-transferase is an enzyme critical to the detoxification and disposal of unwanted chemicals, which carcinogens preeminently are.

- Colon cancer, one of the big three cancer killers in America, has also been investigated. Aberrant crypt foci—those are cells lining the walls of the colon that are growing too rapidly—are common precursors of colon cancer. Scientists found that rodents dosed with a common carcinogen subsequent to being given the garlic sulfur compound S-allyl cysteine had from one third to one half less aberrant foci than did rodents not so protected. The protective effect may have been partly due to an increase in production of powerful detoxifying enzymes.

THE MIGHTY CLOVE

After reading such a formidable array of evidence for garlic's cancer preventive effects, it might seem almost superfluous to rave about its other qualities—that is, it would if they weren't so profoundly significant. Even my devotion to preventing cancer does not blind me to the fact that cardiovascular disease is still the biggest cause of death in America.

Medical research certainly seems to be showing that garlic is therapeutically more effective than a whole host of heart and blood pressure medications that travel in company with a grim panoply of side effects a lot more debilitating than occasional bad breath. A meta-analysis (a sort of summary review of past studies) that was published in 1993 in the prestigious *Annals of Internal Medicine* concluded that garlic, "in an amount approximating one half to one

Pharmacist's Corner

■ Commercially aged garlic is higher in allylsulfides, one of the ingredients in garlic that demonstrate chemopreventive ability. Wakunaga, a Japanese manufacturer, ages garlic for 1 year; the product is available under the trade name Kyolic™. The dosage is one or two 300 milligram capsules, one to three times daily with food.

■ All garlic supplements seem to be helpful. Two manufacturers who make a high-quality garlic supplement are Solgar and Oncologics.

■ There is no research to date showing an interaction between high doses of garlic and anticoagulant drugs, but patients should be cautious about taking garlic if they are taking warfarin (Coumadin). If you take warfarin, discuss with your doctor any plans to take garlic.

■ Recent evidence shows that liquid garlic extracts lack some of the activity of garlic cloves and garlic tablets and capsules.

clove per day, decreased total serum cholesterol levels by about 9 percent in the groups of patients studied."

Garlic is also a natural inhibitor of clotting. In the mid-1980s, researchers at the Poona Medical College in India found that platelet clumping and fibrin activity decreased in direct proportion to garlic consumption—and these are well-recognized risk factors for heart attacks.

The Indians, in whose cuisine garlic is heavily represented, have been vigorous investigators on the garlic–cardiovascular front. Perhaps the most startling research was conducted by Dr. Arun Bordia, a cardiologist at Tagore Medical College in Udaipur. He took 432 coronary patients who had already suffered one heart attack and divided them randomly into two groups, one group receiving daily supplementation of garlic juice in milk. That group had fewer repeat heart attacks, lower cholesterol, and lower blood pressure, and after three years, there were only half as many deaths in the garlic group as in the group taking no garlic.

As for garlic's antibiotic effects, a good deal of research has shown them to be quite real, but not so dramatically, perhaps, as a bit of folklore from eighteenth-century France. In 1721, during an outbreak of bubonic plague in Marseilles, four condemned criminals were assigned to bury dead bodies. The authorities were perfectly aware that this would save them the trouble of executing the men who, so they knew, would naturally contract the disease and perish. All four survived and credited their immunity to the copious use of a folk remedy for infection, wine laced with crushed garlic. It's possible that had antibiotics not been invented, the surgical care unit in your local hospital would have a smell quite different from anything you've ever associated with medicine.

Do I exaggerate garlic's abilities? I don't think so. This herb is capable of doing just about anything except polishing your car and negotiating a tax refund from the Internal Revenue Service. The bottom line clearly appears to be that garlic, the humble smelly rose, is serious preventive medicine. You neglect it at your peril. I strongly recommend that you incorporate it into your lifetime cancer prevention plan and probably into your cardiovascular plan, as well.

CHAPTER

18

FIBER

---

*"When a man lies dying, he does not die
from the disease alone. He dies from his
whole life.*

—CHARLES PEGUY

Fiber is a pure plant product; and so this is a pure plant chapter.

I know almost all of you are secretly tempted to skip this chapter. *Fiber—ah yes*, you say, *big stools, no constipation . . . yawn.* I'm sure you've had the fiber song sung to you by one set of diet preachers or another. Without getting into the details of various diet plans, the fiber portion of their message has plenty of validity. High intake of fiber has a number of health benefits, not the least of which is a reduced risk of colon cancer and breast cancer.

I know from conversations with my patients that many folks think of fiber in fairly simplistic terms—sort of like a vegetable broom that passes through their digestive tract, ending up embedded in their stools like a bunch of straw. It's a great image, but actually dietary fiber is broken down into molecular constituents on its way to your rectum, like every other food.

Within plants themselves, fiber refers generally to the cell walls that give them their relatively firm and rigid structure. There are also certain other fibrous substances and residues within plants.

We do not possess the proper enzymes to digest most plant fiber, so it does not make caloric or nutritive contributions to our diet. Its usefulness lies elsewhere. Consider the following four points:

- Since a sizable amount of fiber absorbs water, it increases the size, malleability, and ease of passage of your stools. This prevents or minimizes a whole host of physical problems that many people are suffering from quite intensely by the time they reach middle age. I'm referring to constipation, hemorrhoids, and varicose veins, which are largely the consequence of vascular damage in the legs caused by straining to eliminate stools.

- Fiber binds and removes cholesterol and various bile acids made from cholesterol and so promotes a more healthy cholesterol level for the heart.
- Fiber binds up and excretes certain cancer-causing chemicals.
- Fiber helps to stabilize blood sugar levels, a benefit to those with diabetes.

Originally, of course, no one knew quite what to make of fiber. At the beginning of the twentieth century when the refining of white flour was just getting started on its disastrous course, most nutritionists were of the opinion that it was useless. In the early 1970s, however, Denis Burkitt, M.D., a distinguished British physician, began to demonstrate that a long list of ills, from hemorrhoids, diverticulosis, and gallstones to heart disease, colon cancer, and appendicitis, were far more prevalent in societies (such as ours) that had a relatively low level of fiber consumption. Today, this is medical orthodoxy and is so well documented that I doubt that anyone cares to question it.

Pharmacist's Corner

■ Both foods with a high fiber content and fiber supplements can interfere with the absorption of digoxin (Lanoxin), a cardiotonic drug.

■ If taking a fiber supplement, take mineral supplements at another time.

■ If you want to take a fiber supplement, try one that includes a wide variety of different fibers; some fibers decrease cholesterol absorption and other fibers create a better stool, cleanse the colon, and promote bowel regularity.

■ Yerba Prima offers a fiber complex supplement called Daily Fiber. Take four capsules one to three times daily or one heaping teaspoon of the powder up to three times daily in a full glass of water.

■ Always take fiber alone. It can absorb medicine or the nutrients in food or supplements.

In this chapter, I'll give you some sense of the overall benefits of fiber for cancer protection, and then I'll discuss two fibers in particular—the lignans in flaxseed and citrus pectin.

The fibers found in our plant food are cellulose, hemicellulose, lignin, pectins, gums, and mucilage. We obtain these varying ingredients from whole grains, fruits, and vegetables. Some of these fibers are water soluble (meaning they dissolve in water) and others are insoluble in water. Foods high in soluble fiber include barley, flaxmeal, oats, oat bran, citrus fruits, apples, carrots, and beans. Insoluble fiber is high in wheat bran, corn bran, celery, and the skins of fruits and root vegetables. Some scientists now believe that most of the protective benefits that fiber has against colon cancer come from the consumption of water-soluble fruits and vegetables rather than from cereal foods; however, the opposite viewpoint has been more commonly held. We don't need to solve this problem yet. Both kinds of fiber are good for you.

FIBER AGAINST CANCER

Let's look at breast cancer first. Not everyone is aware that both clinical trials and population studies have concluded that a high-fiber diet lowers the risk of breast cancer.

At first, many researchers, believing in the attractive (but still unproven) theory that dietary fat is responsible for breast cancer, surmised that the reason for this association was that when diets are high in fiber, they are almost always fairly low in fat. Now, however, it's beginning to appear as if fiber itself is protective. The case of Finland reinforces that notion. Finland is the rare country where people consume a diet that is both high fat *and* high in fiber. Their breast cancer mortality rate is a great deal lower than in countries like England and the United States, with their high fat–low fiber regimens.

One recent study in Uruguay comparing 351 women with breast cancer with 356 controls (women without the disease) found that, after researchers statistically factored out levels of fat consumption, there was still a strong reduction in the risk of breast cancer among women who ate large amounts of dietary fiber. This protective effect was observed in both pre- and postmenopausal women. The best summary of the reasons, which are mostly related to estrogen, was given by B. A. Stoll, M. D., in the *British Journal of Cancer.* He suggested the following:

- A high-fiber diet reduces circulating estrogens by reducing the recirculation of estrogen through the liver. In other words, the estrogen that passes through the liver is caught and excreted together with fiber.
- Many plants and vegetables contain isoflavones and lignans, which are capable of being converted into weak estrogens in the bowel. These then compete with estrogen for binding sites in the breasts and other areas of the body. To the extent that they crowd out estrogen in a woman's breasts, they will generally reduce her risk of estrogen-sensitive cancers.
- A high-fiber diet is generally associated with relative slimness and therefore with lower circulating estradiol levels. Estradiol is the most carcinogenic form of estrogen. Estrogen in all its forms tends to be stored in fat, and heavier women almost always have higher circulating estradiol levels, with an increased risk of breast cancer.
- A high-fiber diet usually has a lower content of fat and a higher content of antioxidant vitamins, which may protect against breast cancer.
- Diets rich in fiber and complex carbohydrates can improve insulin sensitivity, with an associated reduction in circulating estrogen levels. Remember: complex carbohydrates refer to fruits, vegetables, brown rice, lentils, soy, stone-ground wheat, and so on—not to the nutritionally horrific carbohydrate foods that fill up the middle aisles of your supermarket, including the high-sugar and refined white flour goodies that for many Americans constitute a major proportion of their daily food intake.

These are highly convincing reasons for the often observed association of high fiber and low breast cancer risk. When counseling a woman who wants to lower her risk factors for breast cancer, I always put heavy emphasis on an increase in fiber consumption, the addition of soy to her diet, and maintaining a weight within 10 percent of the ideal range.

AND NOW TO THE COLON

When it comes to cancer, the phytonutrients of this book certainly offer a cornucopia of colon care, yet if you had to do just one thing for your overworked, long-suffering bottom half, the clear and inevitable choice would be to load on the fiber. The main reason that our rectums are inflamed, our guts are in turmoil, and laxatives and Preparation H have glutted the market is that we eat a ridiculously overrefined diet. Do you find yourself excreting hard pellets instead of soft, bulky stools? If that's your elimination description, then sooner or later your intestines are going to rebel somewhere along their 30-foot length.

If your luck is really lousy, instead of just being miserable, you could end up with a cancer problem in your lower reaches—not a pleasant prospect. After lung cancer, colon cancer reaps the biggest and grimmest harvest in the malignancy sweepstakes. A high-fiber diet, however, offers substantial protection.

The way it works is like this: First, fiber, by bulking up stools and decreasing food's transit time through the intestinal tract, also decreases the amount of time that any carcinogenic toxins are in contact with the walls of the colon. Second, it appears that a high-fiber diet promotes a more favorable type of bacteria in the colon that minimize the cancer-causing actions of certain bile acids. Studies in lab animals have also demonstrated that fiber gives protection from the carcinogenic activities of certain chemicals.

THE FRIENDLY FLAXSEED

Flaxseed oil is the most concentrated source of alpha-linolenic acid, one of the omega-3 fatty acids that we talked about in Chapter 7. It is believed that alpha-linolenic acid's cancer preventive effects are particularly vigorous against breast cancer.

Now researchers have learned that a type of fiber found in flaxseed called lignan has its own anticancer effects. Lignans are spe-

Special Pharmacist's Corner

■ Because of the interaction between intestinal bacteria and food it is important to quickly review the role of our bowel ecology:

■ Hundreds of strains of bacteria live in our intestines; some provide great health benefits and others, if they are allowed to flourish, are quite dangerous.

■ Probiotic bacteria, commonly referred to as friendly bacteria, create vitamins and other nutrients out of precursors in our food. In fact, the cancer protective ingredients in soy products, flaxseed, cruciferous vegetables, and fruit often require bacterial fermentation to process them into active metabolites.

■ These bacteria will also create short chain fatty acids from the fermentation and degradation of vegetable and fruit fiber. One of these short chain fatty acids, butyrate, will inhibit a certain gene from turning on and in this way butyrate strongly helps prevent colon cancer.

■ Patients with low levels of intestinal probiotic bacteria who have large colonies of Clostridia bacteria have an abundance of colon cancer-promoting substances in their feces made by these Clostridia bacteria.

■ Studies have shown that high meat intake decreases the number of healthy bacteria in the colon and increases the number of Clostridia bacteria in the feces.

■ There are a number of high quality probiotic bacterial supplements on the market. Antibiotics can kill off large populations of friendly bacteria, and if you, have been on a course of antibiotics you really should reintroduce healthy bacteria to the intestines. In fact, it is a good idea for everyone to take a bacterial culture once in a while, and studies indicate that yogurt may not be a good enough source.

■ Purchase a product that is refrigerated and contains the important bacterial strains Lactobacillus acidophilus and Bifidobacterium bifidum. These bacteria are alive and need food, so make sure that your supplement contains F.O.S. (fructo-oligosaccharides). Each product varies in potency, so ask your pharmacist how to take it.

cial fiber compounds related to cellulose that have been shown to help relieve hot flashes and that have demonstrated antibacterial, antifungal, and antiviral activity. Flaxseed oil has up to 100 times more lignans than does the average plant.

Here's how it works. The lignans are changed in the gut into enterolactone and enterodiol, two compounds that can bind to estrogen receptors and that seem to interfere with the carcinogenic effects of estrogen on breast tissue. Scientists have also demonstrated that lignan inhibits the activity of an enzyme called aromatase that converts other hormones into estrogen. In effect, therefore, lignan seems capable of both blocking the activity of estrogen and lowering the amount of estrogen in the body in absolute terms.

It's certain that we yet haven't heard the end of the flaxseed–cancer story. A recent study of rats showed that flaxseed could inhibit the onset of colon cancer in them. I expect to see some very exciting research findings in this area by the early twenty-first century. Meanwhile, you don't have to wait for any further results. Flaxseed oil is a genuine health food in all the best senses that that somewhat overused term can bear. It will strengthen your immune system, offer you protection against heart disease, and provide you with yet another arrow that you can fire at the cancer demon.

I can think of at least two very good methods of getting flaxseed oil into your diet. You can take it straight, 1 tablespoon per day, or you can sprinkle it on salads or other cold foods. If you're buying it in a glass or plastic jar, the jar should be dark to protect the oil. Refrigerate it. Remember not to heat or cook with flaxseed oil, and make certain the expiration date on the bottle has not passed. (Flaxseed oil is very unstable and easily oxidized.)

THE PECTIN STORY

Nutritional science appears to have discovered yet another cancer fighter in pectin, a water-soluble fiber present in the cell walls of citrus fruits (and most other plants.) When the pectin derived from citrus fruits is modified by breaking down its long-chain molecules into smaller ones that the body can absorb, interesting effects occur in the bodies of animals with cancer.

Briefly, this modified citrus pectin (MCP) seems capable of inhibiting metastasis, the process whereby cancer cells are sloughed off from the original tumor and spread throughout the body. This was first observed in the study of mouse melanomas and rat prostate cells. In the case of the rats with the prostatic cancer, scientists at the National Cancer Institute, a division of the National Institutes of Health in Bethesda, Maryland, found that the occurrence of metastases in the lung—the most common site in a rat for the cancer to spread—was reduced by more than 80 percent.

Why? The method of inhibition is quite amazing. Studies of the effects MCP has on cancer cells in the test tube leads scientists to think that it actually ruins the cancer cell's ability to adhere to the tissues into which they have been transported. When cancer cells roam about the body looking for a new home, they need to find an appropriate receptor site and they need to form a chemical bond when they land. Without our getting into the extraordinarily detailed biochemistry of this "fit," it's clear that certain components of the cell surface, including glycoproteins and lectins, must adhere to their new host. It appears that modified citrus pectin makes this act of adhesion extraordinarily difficult.

To date, no evidence has been found to show that MCPs can also inhibit the creation of primary tumor sites, but these are early days yet in citrus pectin research. Fiber is an absolutely marvelous anticarcinogen, and I want to leave you contemplating the distinct possibility that it could be found to be even better yet.

CHAPTER

19

GREEN TEA

Men occasionally stumble over the truth,
but most then pick themselves up and
hurry off as if nothing had happened.

—WINSTON CHURCHILL

In 1991 a witty staff writer at *Science News* wrote an article entitled "Tea-Totaling Mice Gain Cancer Protection." He was right. Your total tea intake, if it's high enough, could put you in good company with those lucky mice. Tea, particularly green tea, is one of the most potent cancer preventive agents found in the human diet. Two to five cups a day might change your life.

Tea drinking is an ancient human invention, and tea is—next to water—the most widely consumed beverage on the globe. I do have hopes that in this country, the public will discover tea in a very big way. Already, a smattering of tea shops and tea bars are opening across America. People are discovering the wide variety of teas distributed by large importers of fine tea. I talked with the founder of one such company, John Harney and Sons Tea in Salisbury, Connecticut who stated, "Tea is going to be the coffee of the twenty-first century, the way things are going. It's not just that a cup of tea has less than half the caffeine of a cup of coffee, but once people try a fine tea, they don't want to go back to the supermarket teas."

All teas come from the same tropical or semi tropical evergreen plant, the *Camellia* species of the *Theaceae* family. Thus, the leaves for both green and black teas are the same; it's the different processing techniques that determine their color, taste, and chemical properties. Green teas, like Darjeeling and Sensia, are more delicate and mild, whereas English teas are black-tea blends, robust enough for the addition of milk and sugar. (Some studies indicate that adding dairy products to tea inactivates tea's cancer preventive polyphenols.) More than 2.5 billion pounds of tea are produced yearly, but 80 percent of this is black, and the remaining 20 percent is largely consumed in the Orient.

WHY YOUR TEA SHOULD BE GREEN

Green tea is tea in its freshest, least processed form. The tea leaves are steamed to soften them, then rolled and dried. Black tea suffers a good deal more to make its way to your teacup. The leaves are withered by air or heat, then broken so that oxygen interacts with enzymes in the leaf. This begins a process of fermentation that darkens the tea and continues until it is heated to make your drink. Variations in technique as well as variations in the leaves lead to the almost infinite variety of black teas.

Unfortunately, all this flavorsome mistreatment produces major losses in the most nutritionally significant portion of the brew. All teas contain easily measurable quantities of antioxidants and powerful polyphenols with demonstrated anticancer effects. The levels of these items are far higher, however, when the tea is green rather than black—approximately six times as many polyphenols per cup. As for antioxidant protection, let's simply start by noting that 2 small cups of green tea contain as much vitamin C as 1 glass of orange juice. The major polyphenol of green tea was reported at the American Chemical Society's 1997 meeting in Las Vegas to be 200 times more potent than vitamin E and 500 times more potent than vitamin C as an antioxidant.

The real distinction of green tea, however, is in its polyphenolic compounds—flavonols, flavondiiols, flavonoids, and phenolic acids—some of which are really not very widely distributed in other foods. These compounds account for up to 30 percent of the dry weight of green tea leaves. The polyphenols in green tea that appear to be most important in cancer protection are called catechins. One in particular, epigallocatechin-3-gallate (EGCG), is—in addition to being the most potent of the green tea antioxidants—believed to block the carcinogenic effects of a number of infamous cancer-inducing chemicals. Some of the other major catechins in green tea with apparent anticancer effects are EC_2, ECG, and EGC—an alphabet soup that spells only good things for you.

Cancer researchers have been hot on the trail of the catechins ever since a 1994 study in the *Journal of the National Cancer Institute* pointed out that green tea drinkers in Shanghai cut their risk of esophageal cancer by 60 percent if they were women and 57 perent if they were men. Most of these people were drinking 2 to 3 cups of green tea a day. This news caused many a medical brain cell to switch on, especially when combined with a presentation made a few years earlier at an American Chemical Society meeting. Then, it had been pointed out that Japanese smokers who drank green tea lowered their risk of lung cancer by 45 percent, which certainly seems to explain why the green tea–drinking Japanese have both the highest smoking rates and the lowest lung cancer rates in the developed world. Another Japanese study found significantly decreased risk of gastric cancer among people who drank more than 10 cups of green tea daily.

If you're feeling relieved that you don't live in a province in China where esophageal cancer rates are so high, consider the fact that incidence rates in the United States have tripled since the 1970s. Esophageal cancer will claim almost 10,000 lives in 1998 in the United States alone. In 1994, a 10-year study was presented at the General Motors Cancer Research Foundation Scientific Conference held in Bethesda, Maryland. In this study, conducted by the University of Washington Medical Center in Seattle, researchers found they could predict cancer risk by examining cells for abnormal amounts of DNA (called aneuploidy) in biopsies of patients with a condition known as Barrett's esophagus. This condition is caused by chronic indigestion and is a first step toward cancer. It is estimated that 5 million Americans have Barrett's esophagus and 5 percent of those will go on to develop cancer within 5 years. Seventy-five percent of the patients who tested positive for abnormal amount of DNA developed cancer or precancer, compared to none of those with normal amounts of DNA.

I have strongly recommended green tea to virtually all my patients who come to me looking for cancer protection. Because of the Japanese and Chinese statistics, I recommend it twice as hard when the lungs or esophagus are in question.

Here's a case you can't help but enjoy. Richard Dunn, a cabinetmaker from Connecticut, was 38 years old when he came to see me, referred by a chest surgeon at Cornell Medical Center in New York who had recently operated on him. Richard was a career smoker: he started his two-pack-a-day habit when he was 15 years old. Two months before he visited me, he had seen his doctor because of a severe cough that had lingered on in the aftermath of a cold.

Well aware of his recreational puffing, Richard's doc had ordered up a chest X-ray. There in the middle of his left lung was an ominous spot half the size of a dime that represented a small nodule or bump. The results of a biopsy were inconclusive. The possibility of lung cancer was very real, and Richard decided to have a surgeon take the mysterious object out. It turned out to be noncancerous tissue resulting from inflammation.

Richard came to see me two weeks later, vigorously struggling after his recent fright not to resume smoking again. I found out right away that both his parents had been two-pack-a-day smokers, too, and his father had died of lung cancer at age 51. I asked him what effect that had had on him. "Of course, it made me leery of continuing to smoke," Richard said, "but you've got to remember I started pretty young. Quitting just wasn't something I was able to do."

In designing cancer protection for Richard, I had two goals in mind: first, to make it as easy as possible for him to maintain his present abstinence from the killer weed, and second, to load up his body with every cancer preventive agent I could think of. He already had a quarter century of smoking under his belt and, even if he never took another puff, his risk for lung cancer would always be significantly higher than a nonsmoker's.

Richard was highly motivated, and I took care of the first part of my plan by recommending that he try some of the breathing and relaxation techniques that you'll read about in Chapter 20. I knew that less stress not only would make him a happier person but would make it easier for him to deal with the additional stress of quitting an addictive drug.

The second part of my plan was a regimen of cancer preventive agents. I asked Richard to drink 3 to 4 cups of green tea a day and to consume soy in the form of miso and tofu. Then I asked him to juice daily—a mix of two celery stalks, two carrots, one beet, one apple, one serving of watercress, and a quarter head of cabbage. Finally, Richard began consuming algae and grass juices on a daily basis and eating a designer food that contained the various bee products you've read about in Chapter 10.

In the three years since Richard first saw me, his X-rays have remained clean. His exercise ability and pulmonary stamina have markedly improved, and Richard now tells me that getting that lump in his lung was the best thing that ever happened to him. He's probably right.

A REAL RODENT TEA PARTY

Results of studies on tea conducted in humans so far are intensely suggestive but still preliminary. Results of studies conducted in animals—who wouldn't normally be drinking green tea at all—are formidable and highly satisfying to anyone who would like to achieve phytonutrient-driven cancer prevention. They have demonstrated that the polyphenols in green tea give mice protection against all stages of cancer: tumor initiation, tumor promotion, and tumor progression.

Here is a description of a few of the most impressive animal studies:

- American researchers found that in mice, green tea extract taken in water inhibited the development of skin tumors caused by ultraviolet-B (UVB) light. The extract also inhibited lung cancer caused by the consumption of a nicotine-derived nitrosamine.
- Green tea extract in water was shown to inhibit cancer in rodents in such organs as the stomach, duodenum, colon, liver, and pancreas.
- Benign tumors can, of course, often become malignant, and one recent study showed that this process—at least for skin cancer—can be slowed or halted in mice by the application of green tea polyphenols to the warts and polyps that were in the process of being converted to carcinomas.
- Green tea mildly inhibits certain enzymes (Phase 1 enzymes) that serve to activate cancer-causing chemicals in our bodies. For instance, a variety of animal studies have shown that it prevents nitrosamine-induced cancer of the stomach. These are the largest single group of cancer-causing chemicals in

our diet and are especially prevalent in well-cooked or smoked meat or fish, as well as in tobacco smoke.

UP FROM RODENTS

Meanwhile, we continue to see strong hints in human-population studies that tea can only help you.

A 1995 study of cancer in postmenopausal women in Iowa revealed an inverse association between tea consumption— presumably, this would have been mostly black tea—and cancer risk for esophageal, stomach, and kidney cancers. In other words, drinking tea reduced the chance of developing these cancers.

An intriguing report came from Itaro Oguni, Ph.D., at the University of Shizuoka in Japan in 1989. He compiled statistics showing that the mortality rate from total cancers and also from stomach cancer (one of the predominant Japanese malignancies) were significantly lower in Shizuoka Prefecture, the leading tea-producing area in Japan.

Finally, I believe I have saved the best for last. If the evidence of Japanese researchers is to be believed, it may well be that the growth rates of already-developed cancers are radically slowed

---

Make Sure Your Cancer Goes Hungry—Deny It Urokinase!

Researchers at the Ohio State University College of Medicine in Columbus, Ohio, have discovered evidence for why green tea has some of its cancer-inhibiting effects.

When a cancer invades cells and forms metastases, it needs certain proteolytic enzymes to unlock the door for it. One of the most important of these enzymes is called urokinase. Research in mice has shown that inhibition of urokinase will decrease tumor size or even cause complete remission of mouse cancers.

It turns out that epigallocatechin-3-gallate (EGCG), perhaps the most potent green tea catechin, inhibits urokinase more effectively than does any other ingredient in food so far discovered. The Ohio researchers speculate that this is what is really behind green tea's anticancer activity.

when green tea is consumed in sufficient quantities. Doctors at the Saitama Cancer Center in Japan made a study of the survival rates of patients with cancer relative to their green tea consumption. The astonishing results showed that patients who drank more than 10 cups per day died 4.5 years (men) to 6.5 years (women) later than did the patients who drank fewer than 3 cups per day. Relatively few conventional cancer treatments claim comparable statistical impact.

GREEN TEA IS NOT SIMPLY A CANCER FIGHTER

Green tea, the phytonutrient champ, has also been shown to lower cholesterol levels and reduce the rate of stroke, perhaps because some of the catechins make the platelets in your bloodstream less sticky. Platelets are the little saucer-shaped cells involved in blood clotting, and if they clump together excessively they can block up an artery, causing a heart attack or stroke. Another benefit is green tea's antioxidant power, which is so great that lab work has shown that it is 200 times more effective than vitamin E. Tea polyphenols

Pharmacist's Corner

■ Studies show that adding milk to green tea decreases the antioxidant activity of the tea catechins. Epidemiologic studies show that there is not much difference between tea drinkers and non-tea drinkers in countries where it is customary to add milk to tea.

■ Capsules containing 170 milligrams of green tea with a 90 percent polyphenol content are now available for people who want the nutrient content without the taste of tea. You should take at least 1 capsule three times a day.

■ Green tea does have some caffeine in it. If you have high blood pressure or if caffeine makes you jittery, green tea is available in decaffeinated tea bags and capsules.

■ Drink at least one cup of green tea three times daily.

have also been found to be strong inhibitors of the acquired immunodeficiency syndrome (AIDS) virus replication system. In addition, they possess antibacterial and antifungal properties. In
experimental studies, for example, tea polyphenols have been
found to enhance B-cells, a key part of our immune system. In
Japan, a study was done in which tea was given to the students at
one school, who gargled with it in an attempt to counteract an influenza outbreak that was then raging. The researchers concluded
that it was quite effective and noted that no class in the school was
closed during the outbreak.

What's the bottom line here? We recommend that you drink
green tea without reservation.

CHAPTER 20

STRESS AND CANCER: METHODS OF LOWERING RISK

*Every stress leaves an indelible scar,
and the organism pays for its survival
after a stressful situation by becoming
a little older.*

—HANS SELYE

In good times and in bad, we've all experienced stress—and wished it would go away. Sooner or later, we notice a consistent pattern. Stress may change—it may become better or worse depending on circumstances—but it never really vanishes. The normal course of daily living creates a considerable number of dark and uncomfortable moments that all too frequently get strung together like a calamitous chain of black pearls.

The real question becomes: What are you going to do about stress—how are you going to live with it? If you don't evolve an adjustment that minimizes its impact on your spirit and your flesh, then you will certainly pay a heavy price. Just in a physical sense, one can say that the effects of long-term and uncontrolled stress are pretty dire. When the body releases powerful stress hormones, like the corticosteroids, immune function is suppressed.

This is not theoretical. People who are under severe psychological pressure have measurably impaired immune systems. Men and women who have lost a spouse or a child, people who are suffering from a severe illness and who fear the worst, those whose financial affairs have gone totally awry—these are people who are very much at risk for fresh catastrophe of the purely physical sort. Statistics bear this out. In the aftermath of severe psychological trauma, people have a significantly increased probability of suffering heart attacks or other ills, including cancer.

It has also been shown that people who are recovering from cancer treatment have better health, a longer survival time, and greater likelihood of not suffering a relapse if they have extensive human contact, including group therapy, or if they have religious or philosophical values that anchor their lives and presumably help to lower stress.

CONTACT THE ESSENTIAL YOU

I once wrote a book, *Healing Essence,* largely devoted to getting in touch with your inner self—your essence. If you can make such contact with your true inner core, then you will see yourself and your place in the total scheme of things afresh, and the difficulties and tragedies of life will become more bearable.

I regret that there isn't space in these pages to properly explore this subject. What I'd like to do, however, is to briefly describe the techniques of yoga and meditation. Most people find them extremely helpful. In fact, I doubt that I've ever met a person who, having learned one of these techniques, subsequently preferred to abandon it.

YOGA

Yoga is a series of physical exercises that had their origins in the ancient Vedas, which were the original sacred texts of the Hindus. First recorded between 1000 and 3000 B.C., yoga aims at quieting the mind through breath and postures. You certainly do not have to be a Hindu to take advantage of these techniques. Anyone who has practiced them will tell you that the breathing, movement, and postures used in yoga results in improved strength and range of motion and increased concentration and energy.

Dr. Dean Ornish's very successful program for reversing heart disease uses yoga in addition to nutritional therapies for reducing coronary artery blockage. I believe yoga gives similar benefits in the prevention and possibly the treatment of cancer.

The most common type of yoga taught in the United States is hatha yoga. In practicing it, one learns various postures (Asanas) such as forward and backward bends, as well as breath control (Pranayama). These physical movements increase relaxation and release tensions from the body and the mind. To learn yoga, get a practical handbook of the various techniques; I strongly urge you to do so. Better yet, find a skilled practitioner of this ancient art who can teach you the breathing and bending exercises, as well as something of the philosophy behind them. I have done this myself and can personally attest to the fact that yoga well taught is a marvelous instrument of psychic and physical regeneration. I don't even wish to imagine my life without it.

DOING A SIMPLE MEDITATION

When you are tense and filled with stress, what do you find inside yourself? Very often, you find more stress and tension, not infrequently combined with aggression, hostility, and paranoia. But what is really inside you? If you could get down to the core of your being, you would find that it is filled with love, tolerance, forgiveness, and compassion. This, I believe, is our natural state.

Meditating is really designed to do no more than bring us back to that state.

Here is a simple meditation—probably best done early in the morning or late at night before you go to bed—that you might like to try. It is in the form of a breathing exercise.

Go to a quiet room where you will be free from interruptions. Sit for a while to calm yourself and lower your pulse rate. Now take some slow, deep breaths in through your nose and out through your mouth with your eyes closed. You should breathe very deeply down into the center of your abdomen. You want to feel the breath coming and going. Remind yourself that breathing is the first and most basic evidence that you're alive.

While you are breathing, picture in your mind's eye that each breath is a waterfall. Imagine that water as flowing down into a clear mountain lake, and visualize that lake as located in the upper part of your abdomen or your solar plexus. Continue to breathe very deeply and focus on your breath.

When thoughts flash into your mind and disturb your meditation, notice them, classify them perhaps as family or job related, and then bring your attention back to your breathing and to the image of the waterfall flowing into the lake. Begin to think about the stress-related tension in your body. Where is that stress? How do you feel it in your body? Where do you hold the tension most?

As you continue the exercise, visualize your body encompassed in a white light. Picture that white light continuously expanding. As you continue with your eyes shut, breathing deeply, imagine your breath filling you up entirely with white light. If you look now, you will begin to see how small that tension is in this immensity of white light.

If you practice this exercise daily, you will begin to notice that stress occupies a less commanding place in your life.

There are many other forms of meditation, but they go beyond the scope of this book. If you're interested, you might want to make inquiries about visualization and imagery, about mindfulness meditation, and about mantra meditation. My first book, *Healing Essence*, is an excellent resource.

EFFECTS OF STRESS REDUCTION

I have treated many cancer patients who felt that stress reduction made a dramatic difference in the way they felt and in their ability to deal with their illness. One of the more interesting cases was that of Vincent Pagollio, a 62-year-old man referred to me by a urologist at New York Hospital, had a 3-year history of early-stage bladder cancer. When these cancers are recurrent, they frequently invade deeper and deeper into the bladder and eventually develop into metastatic bladder cancer, which is often fatal.

Vincent was overweight and a former smoker. He had a managerial job with a large construction supply manufacturer on Long Island. The work was torturous with stress. The company had been downsized several times in the past decade. Four years earlier during the last downsizing, Vincent's position was eliminated. The company then offered him another job with less pay. He felt compelled to accept it.

Not only was this hard on Vincent's self-esteem, but ever since, his wife had berated him for not being assertive enough and for not making enough money. It was no exaggeration to say that Vincent was miserable at home and miserable at work.

I had him begin a series of meditation and guided imagery exercises. I had to work with Vincent so that he could change his perspective and see that he was much greater than what he did in life. I wanted him to see where his power really lay, that it would be found in his essence or his core and not in the man who went to work and who had—or perhaps hadn't—made the right decisions over the years. Vincent was much more than just a work tool. Once he understood that, he would be able to banish much of the stress that was devouring his life. He also changed his nutritional regimen to include fruits, vegetables, antioxidants, and B vitamins. He received a 6-month course of immunotherapy from his urologist.

I reviewed with him the 1994 study from the *Journal of Urology* in which men with early-stage bladder cancer were treated with BCG, a vaccine used to enhance immune function, installed into the bladder. One group was treated with BCG alone and the other also received supplements of vitamins A, C, E and B_6. Eighty percent of the men treated with BCG alone had recurrent cancer, in contrast to only 40 percent of those receiving BCG and vitamin supplements.

The treatment was successful in more ways than one. Over the next six months, Vincent showed no evidence of the recurrence of his bladder carcinoma. Three years have passed since, and the cancer has not returned. Was this the result of stress reduction or was it the result of all the good things I also had him put in his diet? I think the answer is both, but I believe that if Vincent had continued under the dreadful whiplash of stress that seemed at that time to be his fate, no measure of dietary change would have sufficed. Vincent has also been seeing a marriage counselor together with his wife and reports that their marriage is immeasurably improved.

It is very difficult to prove in any individual case that uncontrolled stress causes cancer or that putting a lid on stress cures it, but most of the evidence gathered statistically seems to show that long-term stress is a savage enemy to your health. I think you should add stress to your list of cancer-causing agents and make serious, nonstressful, life-enhancing efforts to deal with it.

THE COMPLETE CANCER PREVENTION PLAN

*Let food be your medicine and your
medicine be your food.*

—HIPPOCRATES

Our complete anticancer plan is based on a simple well-established premise: cancer is seldom the result of one event; it is the product of innumerable actions and choices that occur over a lifetime. Cancer seems mysterious only because, coming often without warning, it can strike the young and apparently healthy as well as the old and debilitated. This mystery, however, is based enitrely on our lack of knowledge. If we could see what was happening inside us during the years—or more often decades—that preceded the moment when the cancer first appeared, we would be able to watch its progress. It would then be robbed of all its mystery and would not seem inevitable.

Cancer, in fact, is often a simple, mechanical, quantitative process. The body suffers so many millions of toxic insults. Like a city under siege, it either has or doesn't have sufficient defenders to protect it from this invading horde. In this great city's beginnings, in its high and hopeful youth, it is most often very strong. It has sturdy walls and thick gates and a plentiful supply of enthusiastic citizen-soldiers who vigorously thrust the carcinogenic attackers down into the ditch below where the macrophage alligators and the natural killer cell crocodiles snap them up.

You must endure this toxic siege for a lifetime. It makes no sense to think you don't need the best defense possible. You do need it. In a situation of such peril, I believe you ought to aim to protect yourself every day in every way you can.

You already know that one of every two men and one of every three women get cancer in their lifetime. Obviously, that fact makes you about 1 million times more likely to get a malignant tumor than you are to win the lottery. Sorry—I didn't mean to depress you, but there it is.

I've seen remarkable changes in people who started organizing

---

Seven Tips for Colon Cancer Prevention

- Consume 1,000 milligrams of calcium daily (check with your doctor if you have a history of kidney stones).
- Exercise for at least 30 minutes daily.
- Avoid obesity.
- Eat a diet high in fiber.
- Eat no more than 2 servings of red meat weekly.
- Supplement with at least 200 international units of vitamin E and 500 milligrams of vitamin C daily.
- Eat such natural cycloxygenase-2 (COX-2) inhibitors as curry (curcumin), resveratrol (red grapes), bee propolis, cold water fish, and rosemary.

---

their physical and mental life along different lines. I've watched their bodies change and their minds become more tranquil, and the changes that I've witnessed have surely—if the hundreds of medical studies that you've read about in this book are any guide at all—decreased their likelihood of ever having to deal with cancer.

Perhaps my best patients are those who come to me with a highly developed fear of the disease. That fear may be reasonable or it may be extreme, but it certainly motivates them to listen.

Take the following case. Marianne Wolder came to see me

Seven Tips for Breast Cancer Protection

- Avoid alcohol.
- Bring olive oil into your diet in a big way.
- Eat soy.
- Supplement with coenzyme Q_{10} (CoQ_{10})—approximately 100 milligrams daily.
- Lower your intake of polyunsaturated fatty acids; be especially wary of hydrogenated oils, including margarine.
- Eat fatty cold-water fish regularly; take omega-3 fish oils supplementally.
- Take at least 100 international units of vitamin E daily.
- Avoid simple carbohydrates such as white bread, cake, and candy.

three years ago, when she was 34 years old, complaining of persistent fatigue. Since a medical workup revealed no apparent cause, it looked as if her condition might be stress related. I didn't have to look far for the source. After a 2½-year battle, Marianne had recently lost her middle son to a brain tumor at the age of nine. Her pain was a palpable aura the moment she entered a room.

I worked hard to convince Marianne that this was not her or anyone else's fault but unfortunately a part of life. I think eventually she, too, came to regard her son's tragedy in that light, and she then expressed to me her fierce determination to see that this never happened again. She wanted specifics about what she could do to minimize the risks of cancer for her family and herself.

I asked her about her life and her diet. She was a receptionist for a large insurance company, and her husband was a sales representative who was frequently on the road. They ate primarily packaged food because "I can't seem to find the time to cook." Rather than simply saying to Marianne, "Eat a lot of fruits and vegetables," I decided to give her a simple 11-point list that went like this:

- Make sure everyone in your family eats 1 apple a day. I talked with Marianne about the flavonoids it contains and suggested that she might want to put other flavonoid-rich foods, such as onions, bee propolis, and grapes, in their diet every day, too.
- Include foods for your family that are rich in antioxidants. Get a juicer and juice beets, carrots, parsley, and broccoli

---

Six Tips for Prostate Cancer Prevention

- Include soy in the form of soy milk, miso, and tofu in your diet daily.
- Eat 2–4 servings of green peas weekly.
- Eat baked beans regularly.
- Eat garlic—if possible, two to four times weekly.
- Eat 2–4 tomatoes weekly (and if you like tomato sauce, choose that preferentially because it has more cancer-fighting nutritional value.
- Supplement with 200 international units of vitamin E daily.

together; make sure everyone drinks at least 1 glass a day. Vary the ingredients; have some fun with it. I gave Marianne the basic juicing combinations you'll find in Appendix II.

- Put some rich sources of calcium in the family diet to protect against colorectal cancer. I suggested low-fat and nonfat dairy products, beans, and leafy vegetables.
- Put cruciferous vegetables such as cabbage and cauliflower on the menu every day. This will strengthen essential detoxification systems as well as modify estrogen to a type less associated with cancer.
- Give your family plenty of daily fiber. I told Marianne about soluble and insoluble fiber and reviewed the best sources of fiber in beans, vegetables, whole grains, and fruits.
- Fashion a weekly diet that has plenty of omega-3 fatty acids and fatty cold-water fish, such as haddock, cod, salmon, tuna, and halibut. I suggested Marianne also put flaxseed meal or oil into the daily meal plan.
- I told Marianne to look at a folic acid list like the one you'll find in Chapter 15 (see page 193) and make sure her family got folic acid in their diet daily.
- Eat plenty of garlic—or at the very least, take garlic supplements.
- Make sure everyone in the family is consuming 6 servings of fruits and vegetables every day. I told Marianne that organic food was best but that she had to eat nonorganic food, then she should scrub and wash them thoroughly to remove as much of the pesticides as possible. It's also a good idea to wash organic food as well.
- Eat natural, hormone- and antibiotic-free meat. Be sure to remove the skin of chicken or turkey before eating.
- Finally, eat plenty of olive oil. It is the cooking oil of choice, and many people find they can become pleasantly accustomed to putting it on their salads as well.

Marianne's family has been eating this way for three years now. I think they like their new diet. I know they're healthier for it. What have they done for themselves cancerwise? I think the answer is very simple. They have adopted the most advanced program for

---

Five Tips for Lung Cancer Prevention

- Consume 250 milligrams of garlic daily.
- Take 600 milligrams of N-acetyl-cysteine daily with food.
- Drink at least 2 cups of green tea daily.
- Take at least 200 international units of vitamin E daily.
- Eat curry (curcumin).

---

cancer prevention that scientific research has so far developed. There isn't anything more sophisticated than what I've just described. High-tech pills—"magic bullets,"—are not the answer that we're searching for; we pretty much already have our answer. If everyone in America were eating the way Marianne Wolder's family is, I believe the cancer rates would drop by more than half in less than a decade, and most of the cancers that still occurred would be lung cancers in diehard smokers.

Let me review for you an even more complete anticancer plan than the one I gave Marianne:

Vegetables:

CRUCIFEROUS VEGETABLES:
  Broccoli
  Brussels sprouts
  Cauliflower
  Cabbage
  Bok choy
  Kale

CAROTENOIDS:
  Beets
  Carrots
  Kale
  Lettuce
  Squash
  Spinach

Sweet potatoes
Swiss chard
Tomatoes
Seaweed
Plankton

UMBELLIFEROUS VEGETABLES:
  Carrots
  Celery
  Parsley

LEGUMES:
  Peas
  Soybeans

MISCELLANEOUS:
  Leeks
  Mushrooms

Onions

Peppers

Shallots

Fruits:

Apples

Avocados

Cantaloupes

Red Grapes

Guavas

Kiwis

Mangoes

Nectarines

Raspberries

Strawberries

Watermelons

Animal foods:

FISH:

Cod

Halibut

Herring

Mackerel

Salmon

Sardines

Tuna

FOWL (SKINLESS):

Chicken

Turkey

Fatty acids and oils:

Flaxseed oil

Olive oil

Herbs:

Garlic

Ginger

Ginseng

Licorice

Milk thistle

Rosemary

Saffron

Sesame

Other nutrients:

Bee propolis

Green tea

Lipoic acid

Pycnogenol

Shark liver oil

N-acetyl-cysteine

In an ideal world, I would set about convincing you to eat and drink each of the above substances daily in the quantities recommended throughout this book. I've tried to do it myself and I have found it's not quite possible. Neither time nor the dimensions of the stomach permit.

I could give you some sample meal plans, but I know what the particular choices I would make would naturally not appeal to many of you. Rather, I think you should make your own choices and learn to discover your own tastes in healthy food. To most fully benefit from this plan, you really will need to eat fruit three times a day, vegetables at every meal, and one or two large salads daily. If you ate like that every day, your diet would be more cancer-preventive than the diets of 99 percent of the people in America.

Even I don't achieve this always, or perfectly. The trouble, of course, is lifestyle. Like most of my readers, I live a busy life. I, too, am waiting for the day that a big win in the lottery will enable me to hire a private cook who can follow me around, preparing at least three perfect meals daily.

In lieu of that, simply brace yourself for big changes, and go as far as you can go toward fulfilling them completely. I suggest that you think about what you're putting in your body weekly and strive to achieve at least the following minimal goals:

Eat 6–8 servings of fruits and vegetables daily. This provides you with 42 to 56 servings weekly. From that, provide yourself with:

- At least 4 servings of cruciferous vegetables weekly
- At least 4 servings of garlic, onions, shallots, or leeks weekly
- At least 4 servings of melons weekly
- At least 6 servings of peas or soybean foods weekly
- At least 4 servings of the carotenoid-containing vegetables listed above weekly
- At least 4 servings of citrus fruits weekly
- At least 4 servings of green, leafy vegetables weekly
- At least 4 apples weekly
- At least 3 servings of tomatoes weekly
- At least 3 servings of beans weekly

That makes 40 servings, and, if you're more ambitious, I leave it to your imagination how to raise it to 56. I know that sounds like a lot of food. You're right. A healthy person who wants to be even healthier can eat a lot of food in a week. The amount of phytonutrient protection packed into the food I've just described could make a cancer cell curse the day it was born.

When you consider that a large percentage of Americans don't eat 20 percent of the cancer protective foods on that list weekly and yet it takes most of them 50, 60, or 70 years, to get a cancer, you know just how well protected *you're* going to be if you follow this plan.

LET'S TAKE PROTECTION ONE STEP FURTHER

The phytonutrient bodyguards in fruits and vegetables form the heart of this plan, but I wouldn't want you to neglect the other nutritional champions described in this book. I hope that all our readers will make a genuine effort to develop a taste for green tea. I would be very happy if many of you started using some of the protective herbs discussed in Chapter 10 in your cooking. I can't encourage you too strongly—for the health of your heart as well as cancer protection—to learn to love fish; especially deep, cold-water fish, such as salmon, tuna, and scrod. Three or four servings a week (or more) would be a wonderful addition to your diet.

Then there are the oils. Avoid polyunsaturated oils as much as possible and completely reject margarine and other foods that contain trans fatty acids (including baked goods that contain hydrogenated oils). Try cooking with olive oil. After a while, most people find it delicious. Use flaxseed oil as well (though not for cooking), or simply swallow 1 tablespoonful daily.

Finally, adopt a modest program of vitamin and mineral supplementation, such as we suggested in Chapters 15 and 16.

We wrote this in the summer of 1998. I believe that as of that point, this is the most complete and powerful cancer prevention program that exists on this planet. Go for it. You could have many cancer-free decades in which to congratulate yourself on the wise decision you made.

CHAPTER 22

WHAT THE FUTURE HOLDS

We are what we repeatedly do.
Excellence, then, is not an act, but a habit.

—ARISTOTLE

W̲e have met the future and it is food. Having gone outside our bodies and nature in search of high-tech medicines to cure our gravest ills, we have now made a big loop and come circling back home. Our cures are mostly inside us. The medicines that we require will not work wonders in minutes or months; they must be taken daily for decades. I think that because we have returned to something that seems very like common sense, we are much better off than we were before.

Not only is it likely that the vast majority of us will be able to prevent cancer—if we want to—but we are now, in some sense, in touch with ourselves. Presumably, that is a good thing. I think it's proper to reflect on the fact that we are not machines awaiting the touch of a magic medical button but whole people whose existence and ultimate fate is clearly related to the steady, day-by-day conditions of our entire lives. What we do to our bodies determines pretty much what our bodies will do to us. The future of cancer prevention, then, seems to me to be very bright indeed.

To step back for a moment from the holistic and the philosophical, let me say that clearly, we have also become more aware of the mechanisms of cancer. There was a time not so very far distant when no one had a really clear idea of what provoked malignant cell changes, much less what could be done to prevent them, but much has changed. Having read this book, you know a great deal more than the best-informed cancer specialist in the world did in the early 1980s.

The cancer prevention program that Jerry Hickey and I have described in this book might be called food-derived gene therapy. You can alter the activation or inactivation of your genes by the food you eat. Science has discovered that the body contains tumor-promoting genes (oncogenes) and also tumor-suppressing genes.

Moreover, there are substances in the body—such as the cyclooxy-genase-2 (COX-2) enzyme that we've discussed so often—that turn these genes on and off.

In the years to come, we are going to learn a tremendous amount about these genes, and that will make a difference to cancer prevention that is impossible to overestimate. We already know so much about the foods and phytonutrients that protect us, however, that we can probably secure a cancer-free future for ourselves and our families now.

Not only have the two of us devoted an enormous amount of thought to cancer and the phytonutrients that are suited to prevent it but we have tried to practice what we preach. *Doctor,* they say, *heal thyself!* I am hoping to have done just that, and I know Jerry has similar hopes. We would like to tell you a little bit about how we and our families eat and live, because that will certainly say something about the conviction and enthusiasm that we've brought to this book.

Dr. Gaynor's Story

I have always thought that doctors who believe in their own therapies tend to live by them. There are exceptions, but as you're about to see, I'm not one of them. Here is what I do to strengthen my body and protect myself and my family from cancer.

I start with exercise. Every morning, I go to the gym and do 30 minutes of aerobic exercise and lift light weights. I follow this up with 30 minutes of meditation. Then I go to my local coffee shop, where they've prepared a juice made from 2 celeries, 2 carrots, 1 beet, 1 watercress, ½ a cucumber, and ½ an apple. I suppose you could call it a phytonutrient power drink.

I take a green drink mixed in tomato juice once or twice a day, and I drink at least 3 cups of green tea daily. I eat multiple helpings of fruits and vegetables daily, and I supplement with 300 milligrams of docosahexaenoic acid (DHA) and 200 mg of coenzyme Q_{10} (Q_{10}), as well as a multivitamin, selenium, and vitamin E.

My wife and I eat in a very similar way, and, since she's a superb cook, there's a great deal of variety in our diet. Our one-year-old and seven-year-old sons drink organic milk and eat lots of fruits and vegetables. We all eat natural, hormone- and antibiotic-free beef and chicken. My older son has gotten to be quite a salad addict, a taste in eating that I couldn't be happier about.

Both children take a DHA supplement daily. The baby has some green drink powder mixed into his baby food, and my older son takes his in a milk shake. I'm convinced that all of us are eating in an exceptionally healthy way. I don't believe that I could write books, enjoy a happy family life, and take care of a very stressful clinical practice at the level it deserves if we weren't.

JERRY HICKEY'S STORY

I have two young sons with voracious appetites. In preparing their meals, we try to use primarily organic ingredients. The boys eat fish three times a week, one or two servings of fruit daily, and spinach or broccoli or carrots every day. They have brown rice or beans daily and whole grain cereal or stone ground bread. They take a vitamin supplement, one DHA capsule, a weak cup of green tea flavored with a bit of honey, and at least one glass of organic juice daily: red grape, apple, orange, or a mixture of carrot and orange. They also get plenty of fresh air and exercise.

All of us eat only small amounts of natural red meat, chicken or turkey (with the skin removed.) We only bake or broil. We never fry or sauté. Olive oil is used as a dressing on our salads. The four of us drink green designer food powders in a small amount of juice daily. We grownups consume seven or more fruits and vegetables daily and a variety of supplements. I manage between breakfast and bedtime to down six cups of green tea. We stick to a regular regimen of exercise and meditation.

Eating and exercising like this has convinced me that a healthy diet is also a high-energy, life-enhancing diet. I wouldn't go back to eating the way I ate when I was younger for all the money in the world.

PREVENTING CANCER

Cancer is a terrible disease afflicting millions and killing half a million yearly. That is why in writing this book we have attempted to emphasize the practical and the possible. We know that no one wants to devote his or her whole life to remaining disease free. The cancer prevention plan that works must be a plan that people want to use—and, we hope, can even find pleasurable.

We are firmly convinced that anyone who sincerely attempts to eat the foods recommended in this book will find that most of them are palatable and many of them are delicious. We're also sure that that individual will also discover that the foods and supplements that fight cancer also support health, energy, and fitness. We have not emphasized those aspects in writing this book, but since the human body is a whole, every part affecting every other part, we doubt that you're surprised to learn that one kind of health implies other kinds of health as well.

Believe us: if you follow the recommendations in this book, you will experience a phenomenal improvement in your life, and that improvement will be just as important as never getting cancer.

Appendix I

Cancer Screening

We believe that in addition to striving to prevent cancer, early detection is essential for those of you who get it in spite of every effort. The Strang Cancer Prevention Center in New York where I work has published the following tables, which I fully endorse, that will help you decide how often to be tested for various cancers.

These guidelines are designed for people without symptoms. If you have any disturbing physical changes, any unexplained lumps or bleeding, please see your physician immediately.

STRANG CANCER PREVENTION CENTER SCREENING GUIDELINES FOR WOMEN

Test/Procedure	Age (years)	Frequency
Complete cancer checkup	20–30	Every 3 years
	40 and over	Every year
Clinical breast exam	20 and over	Every year
Breast self-exam	20 and over	Every month
Pap (Papanicolaou) smear	18 and over	Every year
Pelvic exam	18 and over	Every year
Mammogram	40	Initial screening
	40–49	Every 1–2 years
	50 and over	Every year
Digital rectal exam	40 and over	Every year
Stool occult blood test	50 and over	Every year
Flexible sigmoidoscopy	50 and over	Every 3 years

STRANG CANCER PREVENTION CENTER SCREENING
GUIDELINES FOR MEN

Test/Procedure	Age (years)	Frequency
Complete cancer checkup	20–39	Every 3 years
	40 and over	Every year
Testicular self-exam	20–40	Monthly
Digital rectal exam	40 and over	Every year
Stool occult blood test	50 and over	Every year
Flexible sigmoidoscopy	50 and over	Every 3 years
Prostate-specific antigen (PSA)	50 and over	Every year

Appendix II

Juicing

Juicing is a wonderful way to get a fresh, powerful supply of phytonutrients into your body daily. Here are a few combinations that you might like to try:

JUICE 1:
- 1 Celery
- 1 Carrot
- 1 Beet
- 1 Parsley

JUICE 2:
- ¼ Head of cabbage
- 2 Carrots
- 1 Beet

JUICE 3:
- 1 Tomato
- 1 Beet
- 1 Watercress
- 1 Apple
- 2 Tablespoons of wheat germ

JUICE 4:
- ⅓ Broccoli
- 2 Carrots
- 1 Apple
- 1 Cucumber

JUICE 5
- 3 Oranges
- 1 Apple
- 1 Banana
- 1 Teaspoon of royal jelly
- A pinch of ginseng

After you've tried these, make up a few of your own. If you find any combinations that are really exceptional, please write us at the Strang Cancer Prevention Center, 428 East 72nd Street, New York, NY 10021, or E-mail us at: mgaynor@Strang.org, and tell us.

Appendix III

Breakthroughs in Cutting Edge Nutrients

No one knows just where the next phytonutrient breakthroughs will be coming from. The world of plants is full of mysterious substances, some of which we already eat, without knowing their value, and some of which we will be eating. We are interlaced with nature, and our bodies are programmed to respond to its chemicals.

Some of these nutrients will modify the way our bodies deal with toxicity and some of them will speed up the Phase 2 pathways that rid the body of carcinogens; broccoli and spinach, for instance, are good at that. Some of them will scavenge and destroy free radicals that attack our deoxyribonucleic-acid (DNA). Many will actually suppress precancerous lesions and inhibit certain properties of the cancer cell.

Let's take a brief look at a few good nutrients that might rate chapters in books to come.

FUCOXANTHIN

Fucoxanthin is yet another good carotenoid, and it's actually prepared from brown algae. Research has shown that it has anticancer activity in mice. In one study, mice were given a potent carcinogen in their drinking water with the intention of causing cancerous tumors in their duodenum (the first portion of the small intestine). When fucoxanthin was added to their drinking water, the percentage of tumors and the number of tumors per mouse was dramatically lowered.

In cell cultures, fucoxanthin has had an extremely vigorous inhibitory effect on human cancer cell culture lines. This is a carotenoid just waiting for some vigorous research to be done. Some green drinks have brown algae added to their formula.

KLEVITONE

Having vigorously touted the soy isoflavonoid genistein to you in Chapter 8, I'm forced to confess that some scientists would suggest that another isoflavonoid called klevitone leaves genistein in the shade. Certainly, initial test-tube research has found that klevitone is three to nine times more effective at inhibiting breast cancer cells.

Substances in the body called insulin-type growth factors are active in stimulating the growth of some tumors. Klevitone seems to strongly inhibit these growth factors and also interferes with the actions of estradiol, the type of estrogen that is implicated in breast, ovarian, and uterine cancers. Research on this isoflavonoid is in the early stages, but it looks promising.

INOSITOL HEXAPHOSPHATE

Inositol hexaphosphate (IP6) is yet another ingredient found in the remarkable soybean, as well as in corn, rice, sesame, and wheat. A number of studies conducted at the University of Maryland School of Medicine by Abulkalam Shamsuddin, M.D., Ph.D., and his colleagues have shown that the administration of IP6 leads to a lower incidence of tumors in lab animals. Test-tube research has also been done demonstrating that the nutrient can inhibit the growth of human prostate cancer cells. IP6 is now available in pill or powder form, although I think it is still too early to routinely recommend its use.

PROTOCATECHUIC ACID

Protocatechuic acid (PCA), a phenolic acid, may turn out to be one of the many reasons why fruits, vegetables, and nuts are so cancer preventive. PCA is found in almost all such plant foods, and research has found that in lab animals, it can reduce the activity of a whole host of common carcinogens, such as nitrosamines in the stomach and liver and azoxymethane in the colon.

Other studies have shown that PCA can significantly inhibit colon cancer, liver cancer, bladder cancer, and mouth cancer in rats and hamsters:

- PCA is an effective agent in reducing the carcinogenic action of many chemicals. PCA has been shown to reduce the carcinogenic action of nitroquinoline oxide in the mouth, methyl-nitrosurea in the stomach, azoxymethane in the colon, and nitrosamines in the liver. Also, PCA was shown to inhibit cell proliferation induced by the carcinogenic chemicals in these sites in lab animals.
- Azoxymethane was used to induce colon cancer in male rats. PCA significantly inhibited the cancer without causing toxicity.
- Diethyulnitrosamine was used to induce liver cancer in male rats. PCA significantly inhibited damage to liver cells during the initiation phase and inhibited the incidence and total number of liver tumors. This was also true during the promotion phase.
- Rats were administered butyl-(hydroxybutyl)nitrosamine to give them urinary bladder cancer. PCA supplementation significantly decreased

the incidence of cancer and precancerous lesions in both the initiation and promotional phases. Dietary administration of PCA was quite effective in preventing the development of bladder cancer caused by nitrosamine.

- PCA inhibited the formation of cancer in the mouth of hamsters who were given the carcinogen dimethylbenzatracene (DMBA). PCA significantly decreased the number of tumors in the animals' mouths.

Time will no doubt show whether this nutrient is so beneficial that it deserves to be isolated from the fruits and vegetables in which it finds its natural home and administered supplementally.

CONJUGATED LINOLEIC ACID

Conjugated linoleic acid (CLA) is a fatty acid found predominantly in dairy products and beef. Studies have shown that CLA protects against chemical induction of breast cancer in rats. More recent studies have shown that giving CLA in the early weaning and pubertal periods, when breast tissue is developing, was sufficient to help prevent the formation of breast cancer by the carcinogen MNU later in the rat's life. However, there are indications that CLA may be toxic to the liver.

DEGUELIN

Deguelin, a natural compound extracted from the plant *Mundulea service*, has cancer preventive activity. In a study of deguelin's ability to prevent skin cancer in rats, 60 percent of the rats *not* treated with deguelin had skin cancer, whereas only 10 percent of the animals treated with a higher dose developed skin cancer.

ELLAGIC ACID

Ellagic acid is a naturally occurring plant polyphenol with antimutagenic and anticarcinogenic properties. It is found naturally in strawberries, raspberries, grapes, black currants, and walnuts. Ellagic acid has been shown to inhibit chemically induced cancer in the lung, liver, skin, and esophagus of rodents. In Chapter 6, on carotenoids, those beta carotene–related substances that have so much anticancer activity, we discussed how tomato products have such a strong influence on the prevention of prostate cancer. One other food that inhibited prostate cancer was strawberries; scientists reason that it was the ellagic acid in the strawberries that might have prevented the prostate cancer. DMBA is a carcinogen used to induce esophageal cancer in rats. Ellagic acid effectively inhibited this carcinogen from causing esophageal cancer. DMBA needs to be activiated by the cytochrome P450 detoxification enzymes in the esophagus to cause tumors, and ellagic acid blocked this activity.

Research shows that ellagic acid helps prevent cancer by influencing detoxification enzymes in the studied tissues. It inhibits some enzymes that liberate highly unstable toxic elements from chemicals, giving them the ability to initiate and promote the cancer process, and it also stimulates glutathione and other detoxification enzymes that inactivate and remove dangerous substances from tissues, allowing the affected tissues to detoxify reactive intermediates, or the highly unstable elements formed from chemicals by enzymes in our bodies.

Other studies show that not only does ellagic acid affect detoxification enzymes in a beneficial way, such as blocking the activation of carcinogens and increasing their removal from the body, but it does this with very dangerous chemicals such as benz(a)pyrene. It also protects our DNA, the carrier of our genetic material, further helping to prevent mutations. Ellagic acid has a complex chemical structure, and it has been shown that different chemical groups naturally present on the structure of ellagic acid are responsible for its many different activities.

In a study where rats were exposed to radiation that caused a buildup of fiber in the lungs, the antioxidant ellagic acid, along with other antioxidants, significantly reduced the production of elements that build the fiber—the oxidized radical products in the blood and liver that are produced by radiation.

In a study in which carbon tetrachloride was continuously administered to lab animals, liver damage and the buildup of scar tissue in the liver was significantly reduced by giving the lab animals ellagic acid supplementation.

The nitrosamine known as NNK is a potent environmental carcinogen generated during tobacco processing and while smoking. Some of the enzymes in the detoxifying enzyme system family known collectively as cytochrome P450 enzymes change NNK and increase its toxicity and ability to mutate cells. Ellagic acid helped prevent the P450 enzymes from metabolizing NNK into its more dangerous metabolites.

Aflatoxin is a potent mutagen found on rancid peanuts and corn. In a cellular study, ellagic acid prevented aflatoxin from mutating cells when they were incubated together.

Appendix IV

Exercise

Almost every health book mentions exercise. I don't want to neglect it either. Moving your muscles may sound unrelated to cancer avoidance, but it actually isn't. For reasons that are still obscure, exercise has definitely been associated with a diminished risk of cancer. Some of this association may have to do with the fact that people who exercise tend to have a healthier lifestyle overall. They frequently eat a relatively phytonutrient rich diet, they often weigh less (and overweight is associated with a number of common cancers), and I wouldn't be at all surprised if the portion of the population that exercises the most also tends to smoke the least. Most of us who study cancer, however, have a strong intuitive sense that exercise is doing something else as well. In any event, some of the associations between lots of exercise and a low cancer rate are so strong that I would feel downright remiss if I didn't urge you to get off the couch.

Just to give you a brief taste of the literature, here are two studies that remain eye openers:

- In 1995, it was reported that a study of 6,000 women with breast cancer and 9,000 controls in Maine, Massachusetts, New Hampshire, and Wisconsin showed a modest reduction in the risk of breast cancer among women who had exercised strenuously in their teen years. Those who exercised vigorously at least once a day in their adult life, however, had a startling 50 percent reduction in their risk.
- Also in 1995, it was reported that a study that evaluated 47,000 male professionals between 40 and 75 years of age found that physical activity was inversely associated with the risk of colon cancer. That is, those who were more active had a lower incidence of cancer. The study also found that obesity, particularly abdominal obesity, was strongly associated with a high risk of colon cancer.

HOW TO DO IT

You could, of course, join a health club or go to your local bookstore and stock up on some exercise books. Those of you who want the simplest plan of

271

all might consider walking. Walking is a low-risk, high-yield exercise that almost anyone can engage in. After all:

- You already know how to do it.
- You can ratchet up the amount and the intensity of your walking by slow and relatively painless stages.
- If you don't want to make a spectacle of yourself bouncing around the gym or attempting—after a 30- or 40-year time out—to get back into sports, you can always go out walking, and nobody will even know you're exercising.

Basically, if you can accustom yourself to 30 minutes of brisk walking daily, you will be light-years beyond the exercise level of your average fellow citizen. As a result, you will very significantly lower your risk of heart disease, cancer, diabetes, and a number of other less atrocious but far from delightful illnesses.

You may want to try something a bit more ambitious than walking. In that case, both aerobic and anaerobic exercise is good for you.

Aerobic exercise is any exercise that challenges your heart rate and increases your oxygen consumption. Walking is a very mild aerobic exercise. Running, swimming, speed walking, rowing, bicycling, aerobic dancing, and skiing are all much more vigorously aerobic. Get into them cautiously. If you're over 35, have a physical checkup before you start. Learning to do warm-up exercises will help you avoid injury. That being said, the advantages of such exercise are immense. Every cell in your body requires a constant supply of oxygen. If you've been languishing in front of the television set for years, many of these cells have been making do on short rations. A reasonable amount of vigorous exercise will have remarkably positive effects on your long-term health.

Anaerobic exercise—any form of exercise that isn't significantly aerobic—is also useful. Many forms of physical labor are anaerobic. Weight lifting is a well-known form. In recent years, doctors have realized that such exercise can be extremely health enhancing, especially in the elderly.

HOW TO HAVE A SUCCESSFUL EXERCISE PLAN

Here are a few simple tips:

- Devise a schedule for yourself that you can follow daily. You may want to exercise in the evening after work, or in the morning when you first get up. Whatever your schedule is, it should be something that suits both your body rhythms and the practical necessities of your life.
- Start slowly. If an eight-block walk is hard for you, begin with six. The purpose of your exercise program shouldn't be to punish your body but to gradually develop a level of exercise (it may take 1 or 2 months) that you can live with.

- Use normal prudence. If you haven't exercised in many years or if you're very overweight, start with walking. That will be challenging enough and highly beneficial. More vigorous exercise should produce a normal elevation of your pulse rate. If you feel dizzy or have chest pain, stop immediately. It's time to consult your physician.

Exercise is tremendously health enhancing. I hope you'll indulge. That's the secret about exercise: it is an indulgence. Once you get used to it, you'll wonder how you lived without it.

Appendix V

Resources

The following is a list of recommended supplement and resource companies which the reader may contact for information about cancer preventive products and where to obtain them.

Allergy Resource Group
30806 Santana Street
Hayward, CA 94544
800-545-9960
510-487-8526

Barlean's Organic Oils
800-445-3529

Biometrics
New York, NY 10017
800-724-5566

Collagen Plus
71-777 San Jacinto Drive, Suite 207
Rancho Mirage, CA 92770
888-523-3111

Earthrise Company
424 Payran Street-SP
Petaluma, CA 94952
707-778-9078

Enzymatic Therapy
825 Challenger Drive
Green Bay, WI 54311
800-558-7372

The Haimes Center Clinic
7300 North Federal Highway, Suite 100
Boca Raton, FL 33487
561-995-8484
561-995-7773

Inter-Cal Corporation, A Zila Company
533 Madison Avenue
Prescott, AZ 86301
520-445-8063
520-778-7986
http://www.esterc.com

Jarrow Formulas, Inc.™
1824 South Robertson Blvd.
Los Angeles, CA 90035-4317
800-726-0886
310-204-6936

Marine Biologics, Inc.
750 South Main Street, Suite 104
Bountiful, UT 84010
801-294-8610
801-294-6906

Mariposa Botanicals
151 East 30th Street, Suite 601
New York, NY 10001
888-521-5551
212-564-9161

Montana Naturals
19994 Highway 93 N.
Arlee, MT 59821-9212
800-872-7218 or 406-726-3214
406-726-3287
http://mtnaturals.com

275

NutriCology, Inc.
418 Mission Street
San Rafael, CA 94901
888-563-1506

Oncologics, Inc.
1645A Jericho Turnpike
New Hyde Park, NY 11040
800-724-5566
516-616-5770

Scandinavian Laboratories, Inc.
794 Sunrise Boulevard
Mt. Bethel, PA 18343
717-897-7735
717-897-7732 ,
e-mail: *scanlabs@epix.net*

Schiff (Weider Nutrition, Intl.)
2002 South 5070 West
Salt Lake City, UT 84104-4726
800-526-6251

Solgar Vitamin & Herb
500 Willow Tree Road
Leonia, NJ 07605
800-645-2246

Source Naturals®
23 Janis Way
Scotts Valley, CA 95066
831-438-1144
http://www.sourcenaturals.com
Products available at fine healthfood stores everywhere

Sun Wellness (Sun Cholrella)
4025 Spencer Street
Torrance, CA 90503
800-829-2828

VesPro
9710 Rosehill
Lenexa, KS 66215
800-438-4894
913-438-8907
http://www.vespro.com

Wakunaga of America Co., Ltd.
23501 Madero
Mission Viejo, CA 92691
800-421-2998
949-458-2764

Weider Nutrition International
2002 South 5070 West
Salt Lake City, UT 84104-4726
800-627-0627

ANTIOXIDANTS

Available from the following companies:

Biometrics
PRODUCT NAME: Macular Nutrition
A quality antioxidant combination for eye protection.

Jarrow Formulas, Inc.
PRODUCT NAME: Antioxidant Optimizer
CONTAINS: Green Tea, Rosemary, Grape Skin Extract, Freeze Dried Ginger, Beta Carotene, Lutein, Vitamin E, Vitamin C, Silymarin, Curcumin
In tablet format

VesPro
PRODUCT NAME: Antioxidant Maxogenol
For ingredients in this superb antioxidant product, see Maxogenol in the Grape Seed resource.
Formulated as a delicious, chewable caplet.

Source Naturals®
PRODUCT NAME: Plantioxidants™
Botanical Antioxidant Complex
CONTAINS: Rosemary Extract, Hawthorn Berry Extract, Quercetin, and Silymarin
In tablet format

BEE PRODUCTS

Available from the following company:

Montana Naturals
PRODUCT NAME: Montana Big Sky
Bee Pollen—90 capsules
Bee Pollen and Siberian Ginseng—90 capsules
Bee Pollen, Royal Jelly, and Propolis—90 capsules
Royal Jelly 500—60 capsules
Royal Jelly and Ginseng—60 capsules
Royal Jelly in Creamed Honey—30,000mg, 11 oz
Propolis Capsules—500 mg
Propolis with Echinacea Tincture

CALCIUM

Available from the following companies:

Schiff
PRODUCT NAME: Schiff's Menopause Kit
1000mg formulation in both citrate and carbonate.
This product was formulated with Dr. Susan Lark.

Solgar
PRODUCT NAME: Chelated Calcium Tablets
CONTAINS: 183 mg elemental calcium per tablet

PRODUCT NAME: Calcium Citrate Tablets With Vitamin D
CONTAINS: 250 mg calcium and 100 IU vitamin D per tablet

Source Naturals®
PRODUCT NAME: Calcium D-Glucarate
Cellular Detoxifier
Available in 500 mg tablets

CLA (CONJUGATED LINOLEIC ACID)

Available from the following companies:

Collagen Plus
PRODUCT NAME: Collagen Plus
liquid packed in 15 oz bottle
CONTAINS: Aloe Vera Juice, Collagen, Tonalin-Conjugated Linoleic Acid

Serving Suggestion: one tablespoon per day
Each bottle contains 30 servings

Source Naturals®
PRODUCT NAME: Tonalin™-CLA
Each 1,000 mg softgel contains 800 mg of CLA
RECOMMENDED: 3 softgels daily with meals

CO-ENZYME Q10

Available from the following companies:

Allergy Research Group
PRODUCT NAME: Co-Enzyme Q10 with Tocotrienols
Co Q10 lipid base—100mg
Vitamin E Tocotrienols—400 IU
Rice Bran oil
RECOMMENDED: 1–2 softgels

Jarrow Formulas
PRODUCT NAME: Coenzyme Q10
available in 10mg, 30mg, 60mg, and 100mg
For maximum absorption, also available in a proliposome format in 30mg softgels

Schiff
PRODUCT NAME: Coenzyme Q10
available in 30 mg and 50 mg capsules

Solgar
PRODUCT NAME: CoQ-10
60 mg capsules

Source Naturals®
PRODUCT NAME: Coenzyme Q10
Available in 4 different strengths: 15 mg, 30 mg, 75 mg, and 125 mg

ECHINACEA

Available from the following company:

Solgar
PRODUCT NAME: Standardized Full Potency™
CONTAINS: raw echinacea root and leaf extracts
125 mg per vegicap

ESTER C©

Available from the following companies:

Inter-Cal Corporation
Manufacturer of patented Ester-C®.
533 Madison Ave

Prescott AZ 86301

(520) 445-8063

Fax (520) 778-7986

e-mail: *uscan-sales@esterc.com*

For store brand information, contact: http://*www.esterc.com*

Please visit the website for a complete listing of available brands containing Ester-C or contact Inter-Cal for information.

NutriCology, Inc.

PRODUCT NAME: Esterol with Ester C©

CONTAINS: Ester C® (675 mg per capsule), Calcium (75 mg), Quercetin bioflavanoid (25 mg), Rutin bioflavonoid (50 mg), Proanthocyanidins (2.5 mg)

RECOMMENDED: 2–4 caps per day

PRODUCT NAME: Ester C® Magnesium

CONTAINS: Ester C® (500 mg per cap), Magnesium (35 mg)

RECOMMENDED: 2–4 caps per day

FISH OIL, ESSENTIAL FATTY ACIDS

Available from the following companies:

Allergy Resource Group

PRODUCT NAME: DHA

Fish oil derived from toxic-free tuna

CONTAINS: eicosapentaenoic acid (EPA) and docosahexaenoic acid (DHA)

Schiff

EPA and DHA softgels

Solgar

PRODUCT NAME: Omega-3 700

CONTAINS: eicosapentaenoic acid (EPA) and docosahexaenoic acid (DHA)

FLAXSEED OIL

Available from the following company:

Schiff

PRODUCT NAME: Flaxseed Oil

1000 mg of organic, cold pressed opaque softgels

GARLIC

A full range of garlic products is offered by Wakunaga of America Co., Ltd.

Call 800-421-2998 for information

GINGER ROOT

Available from the following company:

Solgar

PRODUCT NAME: Full Potency™

CONTAINS: 520 mg per vegicap

GLUTAMINE

Available from the following companies:

Allergy Resource Group
PRODUCT NAME: PermAvite
CONTAINS: L-Glutamine (2500 mg per tablespoon), N-acetyl Glucosamine (125 mg), Epithelium Growth Factor (50 mg)
RECOMMENDED: 1–2 tablespoons per day

Jarrow Formulas, Inc.
PRODUCT NAME: L-Glutamine
Available in 750 mg caps, 1000 mg tabs, 4 oz, 8 oz, 750 gm and 1000 gm powders

Weider
PRODUCT NAME: American Body Building
Glutamine
400 mg in powder form

GLUTATHIONE

Available from the following company:

Allergy Resource Group
PRODUCT NAME: Thiodox—Combination Product

Jarrow Formulas
PRODUCT NAME: Glutathione
Available in a 500 mg capsule—60 count
CONTAINS: Glutathione, N-Acetyl-L-Cysteine, Lipoic Acid
In capsule form

GRAPE SEED EXTRACT

Available from the following companies:

Schiff
Available in 50 and 100 mg capsules

Vespro
PRODUCT NAME: Maxogenol
A sustained action antioxidant complex with Co-Q6-10 and Tocotrienols. Formula also includes billberries, rosemary, polyphenols, and catechins from green tea. Formulated as a delicious, chewable caplet.
Each caplet contains:
40 mg Activity White Pine (85% Proanthocyanidin Activity)
45 mg Activity Grape Seed (95% Proanthocyanidin Activity)
50 mg Activity Grape Skin

GREEN FOODS

Available from the following companies:

NutriCology, Inc.
PRODUCT NAME: ProGreens with Advanced Probiotic Formula
CONTAINS: organic gluten-free barley, wheat, alfalfa grasses, Spirulina and Chlorella
Dairy-free probiotic cultures
RECOMMENDED: 1 tablet per day

Oncologies, Inc.
PRODUCT NAME: Theragreens I.P.P.
Designer food containing essential scientifically tested phytonutrients, antioxidants and vitamins

GREEN TEA

Available from the following companies:

Jarrow Formulas™
PRODUCT NAME: Green Tea 5:1
Water extracted, consisting of 50% polyphenols, including 30% catechins
Available in 500 mg capsules and powder form

Source Naturals®
PRODUCT NAME: Green Tea Extract
Contains 100 mg of standardized patented Polyphenon 60™ Green Tea Extract, providing at least 65 mg of polyphenols

IP₆ (CELL FORTE WITH IP₆™)

Available from the following company:

Enzymatic Therapy
Each capsule contains 400mg of IP₆ and 110mg of Inositol
Best taken on an empty stomach

LIQUID SHARK CARTILAGE-CAR T CELL

Available from the following company:

Allergy Research Group
Polypeptides of shark cartilage
RECOMMENDED: 1 vial taken sublingually per day

ISOFLAVONES

Available from the following companies:

Allergy Resource Group
PRODUCT NAME: Ultra Isoflavones
RECOMMENDED: 1–2 dropperfuls per day

Schiff
PRODUCT NAME: Soy Isoflavones Complex
Formulated with Dr. Susan Lark, contains 50 mgs of soy isoflavones. It is balanced with the naturally occurring isoflavones, genistein and daidzein. It also contains other supporting herbs such as red clover, Ginger, and Bioperine.

Schiff also has Women's Natural Replacement, which contains pure soy protein isolate powder guaranteed to contain 30 mg of isoflavones, genistein and daidzein.

Solgar
PRODUCT NAME: Super Concentrated Isoflavones Tablets
CONTAINS: Soy Isoflavones extract—36 mg Isoflavones.
Also contains Genistein, Diadzein, Glycitein and Soy Saponins

LIPOIC ACID (ALPHA LIPOIC ACID)

Available from the following companies:

Allergy Resource Group
PRODUCT NAME: Thiodox—Combination Product
CONTAINS: Lipoic Acid, N-Acetyl-L-Cysteine, Glutathione

Jarrow Formulas, Inc.
PRODUCT NAME: Alpha Lipoic Acid
Available in 100mg and comes in 60 and 180 Quik-Solv™ tablets and 90 caps
Also available in 300 mg (60 tablets) in a sustained release format to minimize gastric irritations
  and blood sugar fluctuations.

Schiff
PRODUCT NAME: Alpha Lipoic Acid
Available in 50 mg capsules

Solgar
PRODUCT NAME: Alpha Lipoic Acid
60 mg Vegicaps®
120 mg Vegicaps®
200 mg Vegicaps®

Source Naturals®
PRODUCT NAME: Lipoic Acid
Available in 200 mg tablets

LYCOPENE

Available from the following companies:

Jarrow Formulas, Inc.
PRODUCT NAME: Lycopene™
Uses a patented emulsion system of phospholipids to maximize absorption.
Available in a 10 mg softgel—30 and 60 count sizes

Solgar
PRODUCT NAME: Lycopene Carotenoid Complex
15 mg Lycopene in vegicaps
Also contains 2,500 IU Carotenoid mix

MAITAKE MUSHROOMS

Available from the following company:

Allergy Resource Group
PRODUCT NAME: MycoStat
CONTAINS: Maitake mushroom and Cordyceps
RECOMMENDED: 1 dropperful per day

MILK THISTLE

Available from the following companies:

Mariposa Botanicals
PRODUCT NAME: Extract Supplement
140 mg softgel capsules

Source Naturals®
PRODUCT NAME: Silymarin Plus™
Available in 140 mg tablets

MODIFIED CITRUS PECTIN

Available from the following companies:

Allergy Research Group
PRODUCT NAME: Modified Citrus Pectin
Potassium base MCP for low sodium content
RECOMMENDED: 3 teaspoons per day

Source Naturals®
PRODUCT NAME: Modified Citrus Pectin—Powder
2 level measuring teaspoons contain approximately 5 grams of Modified Citrus Pectin
Suitable for vegetarians: no yeast, dairy, egg, gluten, corn, soy, or wheat

MULTI VITAMIN AND MINERAL COMBINATIONS

Available from the following companies:

Biometrics
PRODUCT NAME: Ultimate Male
High quality multiple formulation specifically designed for men.

PRODUCT NAME: Ultimate Female
High quality multiple formulation specifically designed for women.

Jarrow Formulas, Inc.
PRODUCT NAME: Multi 1-3™
Fast dissolving, high-potency multi-vitamin and mineral formula. Botanicals added for antioxidants. Iron-free.

PRODUCT NAME: Multi E-Z™
Multi-vitamin and mineral powder, mixes easily and allows for easier absorption.

Schiff
PRODUCT NAME: Regenex
Multiple formula contains a complete range of highly bioavailable vitamins and minerals.
CONTAINS: antioxidants such as coenzyme Q10, lipoic acid, and glutathione precursors.

Solgar
PRODUCT NAME: Omnium (iron-free)
In tablet form

Source Naturals®
PRODUCT NAME: Life Force™ Multiple—No Iron
Metabolic Activator
In tablet form

PRODUCT NAME: Life Force™ Multiple—With Iron
In tablet form

Multi vitamins with a broad spectrum of nutrients, including liver support and antioxidants

MUSHROOMS

Available from the following companies:

Allergy Resource Group
Maitake Mushrooms
PRODUCT NAME: MycoStat
CONTAINS: Maitake Mushroom and Cordyceps (9% total dissolved solids)
RECOMMENDED: 1 dropperful per day

Source Naturals®
Planetary Formulas
PRODUCT NAME: Shitake Mushroom™
Full Spectrum Shitake Mushroom™—With LEM™
Each tablet contains a 430 mg blend of Shitake Mycella Biomass, Shitake Mycella
Extract, Mature Shitake Mushroom Extract, and LEM™ (Lentinus Edodes Mycella Extract)—a
    potent and biologically available form of Shitake
RECOMMENDED: 2 tablets, 2–3 times daily between meals

PRODUCT NAME: Reishi Mushroom™
Full Spectrum Reishi Mushroom™
Each tablet contains a 460 mg blend of two varieties of Reishi Mycella Biomass and a concen-
    trated 6:1 mature Reishi Mushroom Extract
RECOMMENDED: 2 tablets, 2–3 times daily between meals

N-ACETYL-CYSTEINE

Available from the following companies:

Allergy Resource Group
PRODUCT NAME: Thiodox—Combination Product
CONTAINS: N-Acetyl-L-Cysteine (250 mg), Glutathione (200 mg), Lipoic Acid (150mg)

Jarrow Formulas
PRODUCT NAME: NAC (N-Acetyl-L-Cysteine)
500 mg capsules in a 100 and 200 count
Alsoe a 600 mg tablet (100 count) in a unique 3 hour sustain release format for maximizing
    glutathione levels

Schiff
PRODUCT NAME: N-acetyl-cysteine
A precurser to glutathione and L-cysteine
Available in 500 mg capsules

Source Naturals®
PRODUCT NAME: N-Acetyl Cysteine
A precursor for Glutathione Peroxidase
Available in 1,000 mg tablets

PROBIOTICS

Available from the following companies:

Allergy Resource Group
PRODUCT NAME: Symbiotics
CONTAINS: acidophilus group, bifidophilus group, sporogenes, in powdered form.
RECOMMENDED: ½–1 teaspoon per day.

Jarrow Formulas, Inc.
PRODUCT NAME: Jarro-Dophilus
High potency, non-dairy, multi-strain probiotic containing seven strains of beneficial bacteria
  consisting of four different Lactobacilli strains and three different Bifido strains.
Available in capsules and powder.

NutriCology, Inc.
PRODUCT NAME: ProGreens with Advanced Probiotic Formula
CONTAINS: organic gluten-free barley, wheat, alfalfa grasses, Spirulina and Chlorella
Dairy-free probiotic cultures
RECOMMENDED: 1 tablet per day

Schiff
PRODUCT NAME: Milk-Free Acidophilus
100 count

PRODUCT NAME: Nutra Flora
CONTAINS: FOS in powdered form.

PYCNOGENOL™

Available from the following companies:

Schiff
PRODUCT NAME: Pycnogenol
Available in 50 mg capsules

Solgar Products
PRODUCT NAME: Pycogenol® Capsules 30 mg
PRODUCT NAME: Pycogenol® Vegicaps® 100 mg

Source Naturals®
PRODUCT NAME: Pycnogenol®
Proanthocyanidin Complex
Available in 75 mg tablets

RESVERATROL

Available from the following company:

Schiff
PRODUCT NAME: Vinitrol
CONTAINS: resveratrol along with ellagic acid and a high percent flavonoid polyphenol level 60 mg capsules

Source Naturals®
PRODUCT NAME: Resveratrol
Dietary Supplement, Antioxidant Protection
Available in 10 mg tablets

ROSEMARY

Available from the following company:

Schiff
Rosemary extract standardized to 6%
Rosemarinic acid (200 mg) found in Schiff's Glucarate Breast Health Formula capsules

SELENIUM

Available from the following companies:

Schiff
PRODUCT NAME: SelenoMax
TABLETS CONTAIN: 200mcg of high selenium yeast
This was the material used in the Roswell Park Memorial Cancer Center research

Solgar
PRODUCT NAME: Seleno Precise™
Selenium available in 50, 100 and 200 mcg tablets

SHARK LIVER OIL

PRODUCT NAME: Oceana™
570 mg in capsules. See Pharmacist's Corner for instructions on dosage.
Available from the following companies:

The Haimes Centre Clinic

Marine Biologies, Inc.

Scandinavian Laboratories, Inc.

SPIRULINA AND CHLORELLA

Available from the following companies:

NutriCology, Inc.
Refer to ProGreens formula in Green Foods Resource which contains Spirulina and Chlorella

Oncologics
PRODUCT NAME: Theragreens I.P.P.
Refer to Theragreens I.P.P. in the Green Foods Resource which contains Spirulina and Chlorella

Earthwise Company
Call 707-778-9078 to find out where to obtain their Spirulina and Chlorella products

Sun Chlorella
Call 800-829-2828 to find out where to obtain their products

TURMERIC

Available from the following company:

Solgar
PRODUCT NAME: Standarized Full Potency™
CONTAINS: turmeric extract and raw turmeric powder
150 mg per vegicap

VITAMIN A

Available from the following companies:

Schiff
PRODUCT NAME: Vitamin A
10,000 IU softgels

Solgar
PRODUCT NAME: Dry Vitamin A Tablets
10,000 IU per tablet

VITAMIN B COMPLEX

Available from the following company:

Schiff
Vitamin B complex—50 mg tablets
Sustained release B complex—100 mg tablets
Vitamin B6—100 mg tablets
Folic Acid—400 mcg tablets
Homocysteine Protection Formula: contains 25 mg of vitamin B6, 500 mcg of vitamin B12,
    800 mcg of folic acid, along with L-serine, betaine, and choline in capsules

VITAMIN C (ALSO SEE ESTER C© BELOW)

Available from the following companies:

Jarrow Formulas, Inc.
PRODUCT NAME: Vitamin C 1000
1000 mg of vitamin C with 50 mg of Rosemary in capsule form.

NutriCology, Inc.
PRODUCT NAME: Buffered Vitamin C
Hypoallergenic non-corn source of vitamin C
CONTAINS: calcium (450 mg), magnesium (250 mg), potassium (99 mg)
RECOMMENDED: 1 teaspoon per day

Schiff
PRODUCT NAME: Vitamin C with Rose Hips
500 mg tablets

PRODUCT NAME: Sustained Release Vitamin C
1000 mg tablets

PRODUCT NAME: Vitamin C Liquid
Available in 4 oz and 8 oz containers

PRODUCT NAME: Bioflavonoid Complex
CONTAINS: hesperidan, ericitrin, naringen and naringenin flavonoids from oranges, lemons and
    grapefruit.
1500 mg softgels

VITAMIN E

Available from the following companies:

Schiff
PRODUCT NAME: Vitamin E d-alpha tocopheral
400 IU softgels
PRODUCT NAME: Vitamin E Complex
including D-beta, D-gamma, and D-delta tocopherals
400 IU in softgels

Solgar
PRODUCT NAME: Vitamin E and Selenium
Two vegicaps contain 500 IU vitamin E Alpha Tocopheryl Succinate and 150 mcg Selenium

ZINC

Available from the following companies:

Schiff
PRODUCT NAME: Chelated Zinc
50 mg tablets

Solgar
PRODUCT NAME: Chelated Zinc Tablets
CONTAINS: 22 mg Zinc per tablet

SPECIAL RESOURCE SECTION

Dairy
Horizon® Organic Dairy: leading producer of organic dairy products, using no hormones, no
    antibiotics, and no pesticides.
P.O. Box 17577
Boulder, CO 80308-7577
303-530-2711 or 1-888-494-3020
e-mail: *info@horizonorganic.com*

Fruit And Vegetable Cleanser

Organiclean: Naturally derived fruit and vegetable wash made from fruit extracts and an all-natural biosurfactant. (1-888-VEG-WASH) *http://www.organiclean.com*

Garlic

Wakunaga of America: KyolicR Aged Garlic Extract™ is organically grown, 100% odorless, and is the most scientifically researched garlic in the world. For free samples call 800-825-7888; for information, call 800-421-2998

Grape Seed Combination

VesPro: Antioxidant Maxogenol, a super-powerful chewable botanical antioxidant complex containing 40mg Activity White Pine, 45mg Activity Grape Seed, and 50 mg Activity Grape Skin (800-438-4894) *http://www.vespro.com*

Misc. Organic Foods

Graces: 1-888-GRACES-1 (1-888-472-2371)

Natural Meats—No Hormones or Antibiotics Added

Argentine Beef: A natural and healthy source of beef raised on grass. Call Jerry Morelli for product information and availability (1-888-274-2333)

Balducci's: Argentine Beef and other fine natural meat products (1-800-BALDUCCI) *http://www.balducci.com*

D'Artagnan: For availability of organic/free range game and poultry and for location of D'Artagnan retailers, call (800-327-8246) *http://www.dartagnan.com*

Frontier Buffalo Company: Animals are free range. To order, call (1-888-EATBUFF) *http://www.eatbuff.com*

Oils (flax, olive oil, etc.)

Barlean's Organic Oils: Manufacturer of fresh flax oil. Available in healthfood stores. (1-800-445-3529)

Flora: In United States, call 1-800-498-3610.

In Canada, call Flora Distributors, 1-604-436-6000.

In Europe, call Salus Hause GmbH & Co., 011-49-8062-9010.

Carries full line of organic oils, bottled in opaque glass, complete with pressing date. Also carries UDO'S CHOICE® PERFECTED OIL BLEND, an excellent balanced formula of omega-3, omega-6 and omega-9 fatty acids.

Pumpkin Seeds

A wonderful source of natural whole pumpkin seeds and oils:

Helco Ltd.

P.O. Box 69

Mt. Vernon, VA 22121-0069

(800-348-5766)

Wine

Frey Vineyards: Organic wines with no sulfites added. (1-800-760-3739)

Organic Wineworks: Producers of 100% organic wines. (1-800-699-9463) *http://www.organic*

Appendix VI

Nutrients and Patients with Cancer

There is a great deal written today about nutritional approaches for patients with cancer. Although the focus of this book is on cancer prevention, there is much research in progress on developing adjunctive nutritional modalities to be used along with chemotherapy, hormonal treatments, and radiation. The Anne Fisher Nutrition Center is at the forefront of bringing nutritional oncology to Strang Cancer Prevention Center patients. This exciting field brings the best nutritional research to clinical cancer care. Remember to consult your doctor in all decisions regarding your care, however, including any decisions you make about your nutritional intake. The following is a brief overview of recent studies on how nutrients can affect an already developed cancer.

- Researchers at Vanderbilt University Medical Center have found that vitamin E and another antioxidant called pyrrolidinedithrocarbamate induce natural cell death (apoptosis) in colon cancer cells. This effect was found to be due to the induction of a tumor suppresser gene known as p21. Even more interesting, these antioxidants increased the killing of cancer by the chemotherapeutic agents 5-fluorouracil (5-FU) and doxorubicin.
- Researchers at the University of Ohio published a 1997 report in the journal *Nature*, which showed that green tea inhibits the protein urokinase, a protein central to the growth and spread of cancer cells. The lead author, Jerry Jankun, M.D., told the *Columbia Dispatch* about his group's search for an effective urokinase inhibitor, "Some are good, and some are not so good. We published first on this (green tea) because the anticancer activities of green tea are already known and it's soluble in water and is nontoxic."
- A landmark study done by Michael Osborne, M.D., and Leon Bradlow, M.D., at Strang, published in 1994 in the *Journal of the National Cancer Institute*, showed that indole-3-carbinol—a compound found in cabbage, broccoli, and brussels sprouts—has specific antigrowth effects in human breast cancer cells that contain estrogen receptor on their surface.
- Lycopene, a carotenoid, was shown to inhibit growth of breast, lung, and endometrial cancer cells in two studies published in *Anticancer Research*.

291

These studies found that the growth inhibition was associated with a marked slowing of deoxyribonucleic acid (DNA) synthesis as well as decreased stimulation by tumor growth factors.

• Researchers have found that the carotenoids—beta carotene, lutein, lycopene, and alpha carotene—increased the communication between cells. This "junctional communication" is important in regulating cell growth in a normal rather than cancerous manner.

• London's Charing Cross Hospital has been conducting preliminary trials of limonene in pancreatic and colorectal cancer. Limonene is a phytonutrient found in the essential oils of citrus fruits and lemon grass. In animal studies, limonene inhibited both tumor formation and caused regression of existing tumors.

• Researchers have shown that a phytonutrient found in citrus fruits called perillyl alcohol inhibits growth of cultured human pancreatic cancer cells. This compound also inhibited activation of the *ras* oncogene, which is important in the cancer growth process.

• Researchers have also found that the rate of apoptosis (natural cell death) was over six-fold higher in perillyl alcohol-treated pancreatic cancer cells than in untreated cells. Furthermore this study found that this effect was not seen in normal pancreatic cells.

• The most exciting study on perillyl alcohol was done by Stark and co-workers at Purdue University in 1995. They found that perillyl alcohol reduced the growth of hamster pancreatic tumors to less than half of that of untreated animals. Moreover, 16 percent of the perillyl alcohol–treated pancreatic tumors completely disappeared compared to none disappearing in the untreated tumors.

• Several reports have shown that coenzyme CoQ_{10} deficiencies were found in cancer patients. Karl Folkers, M.D., has reported remissions of breast cancer in several patients taking CoQ_{10}.

• A report of a study published in 1994 in the *British Journal of Cancer* showed that patients with breast cancer with low levels of alpha-linolenic acid in their breast tissue were at an increased risk of developing metastatic disease. The authors suggested that supplementation of breast cancer patients with flaxseed oil (which contains this fatty acid) may help prevent or delay metastases. The study's findings are consistent with animal models that have shown that alpha-linolenic acid–enriched diets inhibit breast cancer growth, whereas diets high in omega-6 fatty acids stimulate it.

• A study done at the American Health Foundation in Valhalla, New York, showed that diets rich in omega-6 polyunsaturated fatty acids like corn oil stimulated the growth and metastasis of human breast cancer cells injected into mice. On the other hand, diets containing fish oil, which is rich in omega-3 fatty acids, exert suppressive effects on breast cancer cells.

• Jeanne Petrek, M.D., and colleagues from Memorial Sloan-Kettering Cancer Center in New York reported in 1997 that women with breast cancer whose breast tissue contained high levels of the omega-6 fatty acid, oleic acid, had a significantly higher chance of also having lymph nodes involved with cancer.

• An extract of maitake mushroom was found to have antitumor effects in mice by activating natural killer cells, direct killing of tumor cells, and preventing a decrease in immune function in tumor-bearing mice.

• Tocotrienols (vitamin E relatives) taken from palm oil were found to partially inhibit the development of two types of skin cancer in mice. The mice receiving no tocotrienols had a twofold increase in skin cancer when the carcinogen dimethylbenzatracene (DMBA) was applied compared with those receiving tocotrienol supplements.

• Researchers in India have found that the blue-green algae, spirulina, reversed a precancerous condition of the mouth called oral leukoplakia in 45 percent of patients taking this supplement over a 1-year period. Only 7 percent of patients in the placebo group had any regression of this condition. Within 1 year of discontinuing supplements, 45 percent of the complete responders developed recurrent precancerous lesions. There was no toxicity in any patient at a dose of 1,000 milligrams daily.

• Donald Lamm, M.D., and colleagues from West Virginia University School of Medicine, reported that garlic has "significant antitumor" effects in mice with bladder cancer. The mice receiving garlic supplements had reduced tumor growth, and tumor incidence as well as increased survival compared with control animals. The authors concluded that "the demonstration that oral garlic administration can inhibit the growth of the immunosensitive but highly aggressive murine bladder tumors suggests that oral therapy might be an effective adjuvant to surgical resection."

• Researchers at Harvard University have found that the succinate form of vitamin E (D-alpha tocopheryl succinate) in supplemental form inhibits angiogenesis in laboratory animals. Angiogenesis is the growth of new blood vessels needed for tumor growth. This form of vitamin E also inhibited tumor growth factor alpha and nuclear factor kappa-B, both of which cause tumors to grow.

• Alkoxyglycerols occur abundantly in shark liver oil as well as in human mother's milk. Studies from Sweden have demonstrated that administration of alkoxyglycerols before, during, and after radiation treatment of patients with cancer of the uterine cervix results in higher survival rates than if the radiation treatment is given alone. Also, regression of tumor growth was observed when alkoxyglycerols were administered prior to radiation treatment of patients with cancer of the cervix.

• An Italian study published in 1995 in the journal *Tumori* examined the relationship between nutritional status and tumor growth in patients with non-Hodgkin's lymphoma. The study found in the large series of 246 patients that maintenance of good nutritional status had no deleterious effect on tumor growth.

• A report of a 1994 Danish study published in *Molecular Aspects of Medicine* involved 32 patients with breast cancer involving lymph nodes. These patients were monitored for 18 months in the Adjuvant Nutritional Intervention in Cancer protocol (ANICA protocol). All patients also received standard chemotherapy and surgery. The added treatment was a combination of nutritional antioxidants (vitamin C, 2,850 milligrams; vitamin E, 2,500 international units; beta carotene, 32.5 international units; selenium, 387 micrograms), essential fatty acids (1.2 grams gamma-liolenic acid and 3.5 grams omega-3 fatty acids), and Q_{10} (90 milligrams per day). The main observations were:

• None of the patients died during the study period.
• None of the patients developed distant metastases.
• Improved quality of life as measured by lack of weight loss and reduced need for pain killers.

• A study from West Virginia University School of Medicine found that large doses of vitamins A, B_6, C, and E as well as selenium reduced the recurrence of bladder cancer. In this study, 65 patients with bladder cancer received supplements with recommended daily allowance (RDA) levels of nutrients and 35 patients received high doses containing 40,000 units of vitamin A, 100 milligrams of vitamin B_6, 2,000 milligrams of vitamin C, 400 units of vitamin E and 90 micrograms of zinc. All patients received immunotherapy with bacille Calmette-Guérin (BCG) instilled into the bladder. At 10 months, 80 percent of the patients taking RDA-level supplements had recurrent cancer compared to 40 percent of the patients on high-dose supplements.

• Bosland and colleagues at New York University Medical Center showed that the soy phytonutrient genistein inhibits human prostate cancer cell growth regardless of whether such cells possessed androgen or estrogen receptors on their surfaces. They found that genestein induced natural cell death (apoptosis) in 20 percent of cells compared with no apoptosis in control cells. The author suggests that the genistein induced inhibition of prostate cell growth accounts for the low risk of prostate cancer in countries with a high soy intake.

• Scientists at the University of Milan in Italy examined the effects of genistein with adriamycin (a common chemotherapeutic drug used to treat breast cancer) in three human breast cancer cell lines. Genistein inhibited all three cell lines. The combination produced even greater effects than would be expected from the two added together—called a synergistic effect.

References

CHAPTER 3

Bass, Faye, M.S., et al. "The need for dietary counseling of cancer patients as indicated by nutrient and supplement intake." *Journal of American Diet Association* 1995;1319–1321.

Fortes, C. "Aging, zinc, and cell-mediated immune response." *Aging Clinical and Experimental Research* 1995;7:75–76.

Hannigan, B. "Diet and immune function." *British Journal of Biomedical Sciences* 1994;51:252–259.

Kiremidijian-Schumacher, L., et al. "Supplementation with selenium and human immune cell function. Its effect on cytotoxic lymphocytes and natural killer cells." *Biological Trace Element Research* 1994;41:115–127.

CHAPTER 4

Coscinu, S., et al. "Neuroprotective effect of reduced glutathione on cisplatin-based chemotherapy in advanced gastric cancer: a randomized double-blind, placebo-controlled trial." *Journal of Clinical Oncology* 1995;19:25–32.

Mara, J., et al. "Glutathione and morbidity in a community-based sample of elderly." *Journal of Clinical Epidemiology* 1994;47:1021–1036.

CHAPTER 5

Block, G. *Nutrition Reviews* 1992;50:207–213.

Brown, S., and White D. International Symposium on Pycnogenol, Bordeux, France, October 1990.

Frankel, E. N., et al. "Inhibition of human LDL oxidation by resveratrol." *Lancet* 1993;341:1103–1104.

Jang, M., et al. "Cancer chemopreventive activity of resveratrol, a natural product derived from grapes." *Science* 1997;275:218–220.

Lockwood, K., et al. "Partial and complete regression of breast cancer in patients in relation to dosage of coenzyme Q_{10}." *Biochemical and Biophysical Research Communications* 1994;199:1504–1508.

Tixier, J. M., et al. "Evidence by in vivo and in vitro studies that binding of pycnogenols to elastin affects its rate of degradation by elastases." *Biochemical Pharmacology* 1984;33:3933–3339.

Wegrowski, J., et al. "The effect of procyanidolic oligomers on the composition of normal and hypercholesterolemic rabbit aortas." *Biochemical Pharmacology* 1984;33:3491–3497.

CHAPTER 6

Batieha, A. M., et al. "Serum micronutrients and the subsequent risk of cervical cancer in a population-based nested case-control study." *Cancer Epidemiology, Biomarkers and Prevention* 1993;2:335–339.

Clinton, S. K., et al. "Cis-trans isomers of lycopene in the human prostate: a role in cancer prevention [meeting abstract]." *FASEB Journal* 1995;9:A442.

Di Mascio, P., et al. *Archives of Biochem Biophys* 1989;

Franceschi, S., et al. "Tomatoes and risk of digestive-tract cancers." *International Journal of Cancer* 1994;59:181–184.

Freudenheim, J. L., et al. "Premenopausal breast cancer risk and intake of vegetables, fruits, and related nutrients." *Journal of the National Cancer Institute* 1996;88:340–348.

Kohlmeier, L., et al. "Lycopene and myocardial infraction risk in the Euramic Study." *American Journal of Epidemiology* 1997;146:618–626.

Levy, J., et al. "Lycopene, the major tomato carotenoid, delays cell cycle in breast, lung and endometrial cancer cells [abstract]." *Anticancer Research* 1995; 15:1655.

Mangels, A. R., et al. "Carotenoid content of fruits and vegetables: on evaluation of analytic data." *Journal of the American Dietetic Association* 1993;93:284–286.

Nomura, A. M., et al. "Serum micronutrients and upper aerodigestive tract cancer." *Cancer Epidemiology, Biomarkers and Prevention* 1997;6:407–412.

Palan, P. R., et al. "Plasma levels of beta-carotene, lycopene, canthaxanthin, retinol, and alpha- and tau-tocopherol in cervical intraepithelial neoplasia and cancer." *Clinical Cancer Research* 1996;2:181–185.

Seddon, J. M., et al. "Dietary carotenoids, vitamins A, C, and E, and advanced age-related macular degeneration." *Journal of the American Medical Association* 1994;272:1414–1420.

CHAPTER 7

Caygill, C. P., et al. "Fat, fish, fish oil and cancer." *British Journal of Cancer* 1996;74:159–164.

Rose, P. D., Connolly, J. M., "Effects of dietary omega-3 fatty acids on human breast cancer growth and metastases in nude mice." *Journal of the National Cancer Institute* 1993;85:1743–1747.

Willet, C. W., Stampfer, J. M., Mansor, E. J., Colditz, A. G., Speizer, E. F., Rosner A. B., Sampson, A. L., Hennekins, H. C., "Intake of trans fatty acids and risks of cornary heart disease among women." *Lancet* 1993:341:581–585.

Zhu, J. R., et al. "Fatty acid composition of breast adipose tissue in breast cancer patients and in patients with benign breast disease." *Nutrition and Cancer* 1995;24:151–160.

CHAPTER 8

Bain, R. P., et al. "Racial differences in survival of women with breast cancer." *Journal of Chronic Diseases* 1986;39:631–642.

Fotis, T., et al. "Genistein, a dietary derived inhibitor of in vitro angiogenesis," Proceedings of the National Academy of Science," 1993;90:2690–2694.

Kyle, E., et al. "Genistein inhibits prostate cancer cell growth by inducing apoptosis [abstract]." *Proceedings of the Annual Meeting of the American Association of Cancer Research* 1996;36:A2451.

Lamartiniere, C. A., et al. "Genistein suppresses mammary cancer in rats." *Carcinogenesis* 1995;16:2833–2840.

Monti, E., Sinha B. K. "Antiproliferation effect of genistein and adriamycin against estrogen- dependent and- independent human breast carcinoma cell lines." *Anticancer Research* 1994;14:1221–1226.

Murrill, W. B., et al. "Prepubertal genistein exposure suppresses mammary cancer and enhances gland differentiation in rats." *Carcinogenesis* 1996; 17:1451–1457.

Nutr, J. O., Persky, V., Van Horn L. "Epidemiology of soy and cancer: Perspectives and Directions"[1] *Journal of Nutrition* 1995;125:709S–712S.

Yip, I., et al. "Nutritional approaches to the prevention of prostate cancer progression." *Advances in Experimental Medicine and Biology* 1996;399: 173–181.

Zava, D. T., Euwe, G., "Estrogenic and antiproliferative properties of genistein and other flavonoids in human breast cancer cells in vitro." *Nutrition and Cancer* 1997;27:31–40.

Zhou, Y, Lee A. S., "Mechanism for the suppression of the mamalian stress response by genisten, an anticancer phytoestrogen from soy." *Journal of the National Cancer Institute* 1998;90:381–388.

CHAPTER 9

Bradlow, H. L., et al. "Effects of dietary indole-3-carbinol on estradiol metabolism and spontaneous mammary tumors in mice." *Carcinogenesis* 1994;12:1571–1574.

Chen, I., et al. "Indole-3-carbinol and diindolylmethane as aryl hydrocarbon (Ah) receptor agonists and antagonists in T47D human breast cancer cells." *Fundamentals of Applied Toxicology* 1996;30:183.

Gerhauser, C., et al. "Cancer chemoprevention potential of sulforamate, a novel analogue of sulforaphane that induces Phase 2 drug-metabolizing enzymes." *Cancer Research* 1997;57:272–278.

Haenzel, W., et al. "A case-control study of large bowel cancer in Japan." *Journal of the National Cancer Institute* 1980;64:17–22.

Michnovicz, J. J., Bradlow H. L. "Induction of estradiol metabolism by dietary indole-e-carbinol in humans." *Journal of the National Cancer Institute* 1990;82:947–949.

Tiwari, R. K., Li Guo, Bradlow, H. L., Telang, N. T., Osborne, M. P., "Selective responsiveness of human breast cancer cells to indole-3 carbinol, a chemopreventive agent." *Journal of the National Cancer Institute* 1994;86:126–131.

Yuesheng Zg, Kensler, T. W., Cheon-Gyu Cho, Posner, G. H., Talalay, P., et al. "Anticarcinogenic activities of sulforaphane and structurally related synthetic NorbomyL isothiocynates." *Proceedings of the National Academy of Sciences* 1994;3147–3150.

Verhoeven, D. T., et al. "Epidemiological studies on brassica vegetables and cancer risk." *Cancer Epidemiological Biomarkets* 1996;5:733–748.

CHAPTER 10

Azuine, M. A., Bhide S.V. "Protective single/combined treatment with betel leaf and turmeric against methyl (acetoxymethyl) nitrosamine-induced hamster oral carcinogenesis." *International Journal of Cancer* 1992;51:412–415.

Chiao, C., et al. "Apoptosis and altered redox state induced by caffeic acid phenethyl ester (CAPE) in transformed rat fibroblast cells." *Cancer Research* 1995;55:3576–3583.

Harunobu, A., et al. "Dietary rosemary suppresses 7,12-dimethylbenz(a)anthracene binding to rat mammary cell DNA." *Journal of Nutrition* 1996; 126:1475–1480.

Huang, M. T., et al. "Inhibitory effect of curcumin, chlorogenic acid and ferulic acid on tumor promotion in mouse skin by 12-0-Tetradecanoylphorbol-13 acetate." *Cancer Research* 1988;48:5941–5946.

Huang, M. T., et al. "Inhibition of skin tumorigenesis by rosemary and its constituents carnosol and ursolic acid." *Cancer Research* 1994;54:701–708.

Huang, M. T., et al. "Inhibitory effect of dietary rosemary on mammary and colon carcinogenesis in mice." *Proceedings of the Annual Meeting of the American Association of Cancer Research* 1995;36:A3514.

Huang, M. T., et al. "Inhibitory effects of caffeic acid phenethyl ester (CAPE) on 12-O-tetradecanoylphorbal-13-acetate-induced tumor promotion in mouse skin and the synthesis of DNA, RNA and protein in HeLa cells." *Carcinogenesis* 1996;17:76–765.

Katiyar, S., et al. "Protective effects of silymarin against photocarcinogenesis in a mouse skin model." *Journal of the National Cancer Institute* 1997;89:556–565.

Kuttan, R., et al. "Turmaric and curcumin as topical agents in cancer therapy." *Tumori* 1987;73:29–31.

Lersch, C., et al. "Stimulation of immunocompetent cells in patients with gastrointestinal tumors during an experimental therapy with low-dose cyclophophamide, thymostimulin, and *Echinacea purpurea* extract (echinacin)." *Tumordiagen Therapy* 1992;13:115–120.

Mose, J. R. *Die Mediz. Welt.* 1983;34:1463.

Mukhtar, H., et al. "Inhibition of mouse skin tumor promotion by ethanol extract of ginger root [meeting abstract]." *Proceedings of the Annual Meeting of the American Association of Cancer Researchers* 1995;36:A3535.

Nagabhushan, M., Bhide, S.V. "Antimutagenicity and anticarcinogenicity of tumeric." *Journal of Nutrition Growth Cancer* 1987;4:83.

Offord, E. A., et al. "Rosemary components inhibit benzo(a)pyrene-induced genotoxicity in human bronchial cells." 1995;16:2057–2062.

Polasa, K., et al. "Effect of tumeric on urinary mutagens in smokers." *Mutagen* 1992;7:107–109.

Rao, C., et al. "Chemoprevention of colon cancer by dietary curcumin." *Annals of the New York Academy of Sciences* 1995;768:201–204.

Sarkar, S., et al. *Anticancer Research* 1988;16:1055.

Shibata, S., et al. "Inhibitory effects of licochalcone A isolated from Glycyrrhiza inflata root on inflammatory ear edema and tumour promotion in mice." *Planta Medica* 1991;57(3):2214.

Singletary, K., Gutierrez, E. "Rosemary extract increases liver GSH-transferase and quinone reductase activities." *FASEB Journal* 1993;7:A866.

Singletary, K., et al. "Inhibition of 7,12-dimethyllbenz[a]anthracene (DMBA)-induced mammary turmorigenisis and DMBA-DNA adduct formation by curcumin." *Cancer Letters* 1996;103:137–141.

Stimpel, M., et al. "Macrophage activation and induction of macrophage cytotoxicity by purified polysaccharide fractions from the plant *Echinacea purpurea*." *Infection and Immunity* 1984;46:845–849.

Suzuki, F., et al. "Inhibitory effect of glycyrrhizin (GR), an active component of licorice roots, on an experimental pulmonary metastatis in mice inoculated with B16 melanoma [meeting abstract]." *Proceedings of the Annual Meeting of the American Association of Cancer Researchers* 1997;38:A802.

Wang, Z. Y., Rajesh Agarwal, Wasiuddin A. Khan, Hasan Mukhtar, et al. "Short communication protein against beno[a]pyrene—and N-nitrosadiethylamine—induced lung and forestomach tumorigenesis in A/J mice by water of extracts of green tea and licorice." *Carcinogenesis* 1992;13:1491–1494, 1992.

Vittek, J., et al. "Effect of royal jelly on serum lipids in experimental animals and humans with atherosclerosis." *Experientia* 1995;51:927–935.

Wu, X. G., Zhu, D. H. "Influence of ginseng upon the development of liver cancer induced by diethylnitrosamine in rats." *Journal of Tongji Medical University* 1990;10:141–145.

Yun, T. K., Choi, S. Y. "Preventive effect of Ginseng intake against various human cancers: a case control study on 1987 pairs." *Cancer Epidemiology, Biomarkers and Prevention* 1995;4:401–408.

Yun, T. K., et al. "Anticarcinogenic effect on long-term oral administration of red ginseng on newborn mice exposed to various chemical carcinogens." *Cancer Detection and Prevention* 1983;6:515–525.

Yun, T. K., et al. "Cohort study on ginseng intake and cancer for population over 40 years old in ginseng production areas (a preliminary report) [meeting abstract]." Second International Cancer Chemo Prevention Conference, April 26–30, 1993:132, Berlin, Germany.

Zhand D., et al. "Ginseng extract scavenges hydroxyl radical and protects unsaturated fatty acids from decomposition caused by iron-mediated lipid peroxidation." *Free Radical Biology and Medicine* 1996;20:145–150.

CHAPTER 11

Abe, S., Kaneda, T. "The effect of edible seaweeds on cholesterol metabolism in rats." In: *Proceedings of the Seventh International Seaweed Symposium.* New York: Wiley & Sons, 1972:562–565.

Daigo, K., et al. "Pharmacological studies of sodium alginate. I. Protective effect of sodium alginate on mucous membranes of upper-gastrointestinal tract." *Yajugaku Zasshi* 1981;101:452–457.

Hoshiyama, Y., et al. "A case-control study of colorectal cancer and its relation to diet, cigarettes, and alcohol consumption in Saitama Prefecture, Japan." *Tohoku Journal of Experimental Medicine* 1993;171:151–165.

Mathew, B., et al. "Evaluation of chemoprevention of oral cancer with Spirulina fusiformis." *Nutrition and Cancer* 1995;24:197–202.

Schwartz, J. L., et al. "Prevention of experimental oral cancer by extracts of *Spirulina-Dunaliella* algae." *Nutrition and Cancer* 1988;11:127–134.

Teas, J., et al. "Dietary seaweed (*Laminaria*) and mammary carcinogenesis in rats." *Cancer Research* 1984;44:2758–2761.

Terwel, L., et al. "Antimutagenic activity of some naturally occurring compounds towards cigarette smoke condensate and benzo[a]pyrene in the Salmonella/ microsome assay." *Mutation Research* 1985;152:1–4.

CHAPTER 12

Adachi, et al. "Potentiation of host-mediated antitumor activity in mice by beta-glucan obtained from *Grifola frondosa* (Maitake)." *Chemical Pharmaceutical Bulletin* 1987;35:262.

Chirara, G., et al. "Inhibition of mouse sarcoma 180 by polysaccharides from *Lentinus edodes.*" *Nature* 1969;222:637–638.

Mori, K., et al. "Antitumor activities on edible mushrooms by oral administration." In: *Proceedings of the International Symposium on Scientific and Technical Aspects of Cultivating Edible Fungi.* Pennsylvania State University, 1986:

Nanba, H. "Maitake D-fraction, healing and preventing potential for cancer." *Townsend Letter for Doctors and Patients* February-March 1996:84–85.

Nanba, H., et al. "Activity of maitake D-fraction to inhibit carcinogenesis and metastasis." *Annals of the New York Academy of Sciences* 1995;768:243–245.

CHAPTER 13

Boeyrd, B., Hallgren, B., Ställberg, G., et al. "Studies on the effect of methoxy-substituted glycerol ethers on tumor growth and metastasis formation." *British Journal of Experimental Pathology* 1971;52:221–230.

Brohult, A., et al. "Regression of tumour growth after administration of alkoxyol-glycerols." *Acta Obstetricia et Gynecologica Scandinavica* 1978;57:79–83.

Brohult, A., et al. "Reduced mortality in cancer patients after administration of alkoxyglycerols." *Acta Obstetricia Gynecologica Scandinavica* 1986;65:779–785.

LaVecchia, C., et al. "Medical history, diet and pancreatic cancer." *Oncology* (Basel) 1990;47:463–466.

Linman, J. W., et al. *Journal of Laboratory and Clinical Medicine* 1959; 54:335.

Martin-Moreno, J. M., et al. "Dietary fat, olive oil intake and breast cancer risk." *International Journal of Cancer* 1994;58:774–780.

Strandberg, E., et al. "Variations of hepatic cholesterol precursors during altered flows of endogenous and exogenous squalene in the rat." *Biochemistry and Biophysiology Acta* 1989;1001:150–156.

Studies on the Effect of Methoxy Substituted Glycenol Ethers on Tumour Growth and Metastasis Formation. B. Boeryd, B. Hallgren and G. Ställberg.

Van Duuren, B. L., Goldschmidt, B. M. "Co-carcinogenic and tumor-promoting agents in tobacco carcinogenesis." *Journal of the National Cancer Institute* 1976;56:1237–1242.

CHAPTER 14

Crist, D. M., et al. "Exogenous growth hormone treatment alters body composition and increases natural killer cell activity in women with impaired endogenous growth hormone secretion." *Metabolism* 1987;36:1115–1117.

Fahr, M. J., et al. "Glutamine enhances immunoregulation of tumor growth." *Journal of Parenteral and Enteral Nutrition* 1994;18(supplement).

Hays, S. D., et al. "Dietary supplementation with L-arginine: modulation of tumour-infiltrating lympocytes in patients with colorectal cancer." *British Journal of Surgery* 1987;84:238–241.

Klimberg, V. S., et al. "Glutamine suppresses PGE-2 synthesis and breast cancer growth." *Journal of Surgical Research* 1996;63:293–297.

Ma, O., et al. "Effect of supplemental L-arginine in a chemical-induced model of colorectal cancer." *World Journal of Surgery* 1996;20:1087–1091.

Monroe, W. E., et al. "Effect of growth hormone on the adult canine thymus." *Thymus* 1987;9:173–187.

Moriguchi, S., et al. "Functional changes in human lympocytes and monocytes after in vitro incubation with arginine." *Nutrition Research* 1987;7:719–729.

Muscaritoli, M., et al. "Oral glutamine in the prevention of chemotherapy-induced gastrointestinal toxicity." *European Journal of Cancer* 1997; 33:319–320.

Rudman, D., et al. "Effects of human growth hormone in men over 60 years old." *The New England Journal of Medicine* 1990;323:1–6.

Souba, W. W. "Glutamine and cancer." *Annals of Surgery* 1993;218:715–728.

CHAPTER 15

Block, G. "Vitamin C and cancer prevention: the epidemiologic evidence." *American Journal of Clinical Nutrition* 1991;53:270S–282S.

Butterworth, Jr., C. E. "Folate status, women's health, pregnancy outcome, and cancer." *Journal of the American College of Nutrition* 1993;12:438–441.

Connor, H. J., et al. "Effect of increased intake of vitamin C on the mutagenic activity of gastric juice and intrajastric concentrations of ascorbic acid." *Carcinogenesis* 1985;6:1675–1676.

Corder, E. H., et al. "Seasonal variation in Vitamin D, vitamin D–binding protein and dehydroepiandrosterone: risk of prostate cancer in black and white men." *Cancer Epidemiology, Biomarkers and Prevention* 1995;4:655–659.

De Palo, G., Formelli, F. "Risks and benefits of retinoids in the chemoprevention of cancer." *Drug Safety* 1995;13:245–256.

Enstrom, J. E. "Hypovitamins D in medical patients." *Epidemiology* 1992.

Garewal, H. "Antioxidants in oral cancer prevention." *American Journal of Clinical Nutrition* 1995;62(supplement):110S–1106S.

Garland, C. F., et al. "Dietary vitamin D and calcium and risk of colorectal cancer: a 19-year prospective study in men." *Lancet* 1985;1:307–309.

Garland, C. F. et al. "Serum 25-hydroxyvitamin D and colon cancer: eight-year prospective study." *Lancet* 1989:1176–1178.

Glynn, S. A., Albanes D. "Folate and cancer: a review of the literature." *The New England Journal of Medicine* 1998;338:777–783.

Heimburger, D. C., et al. "Improvement in bronchial squamous metaplasia in smokers treated with folate and vitamin B_{12}: report of a preliminary randomized, double-blind intervention trial." *Journal of the American Medical Society* 1988;259:1525–1530.

Heinon O. P., et al. *Journal of the National Cancer Institute* 1998;90:414–415, 440–446.

Hong, W. K., et al. "13-*cis*-retinoic acid in the treatment of oral leukoplakia." *New England Journal of Medicine* 1986;315:1501–1505.

Howe, G. R., et al. "Dietary factors and risk of breast cancer. Combined analysis of 12-case control studies." *Journal of the National Cancer Institute* 1990;82:561–569.

Hurley, D. "High folic acid intake may cut colon cancer risk by one-third." *Medical Tribune* June 24, 1993;5.

Journal of the National Cancer Institute 1984;1–72.

Kleibeuker, J. H., et al. "Calcium and vitamin D: possible protective agents against colorectal cancer?" *European Journal of Cancer* 1995;31A:1081–1084.

Knekt, P., et al. "Serum vitamin E level and risk of female cancers." *International Journal of Epidemiology* 1988;17:281–286.

Lippman, S. H., et al. "Retinoids and chemoprevention: clinical and basic studies." *Journal of Cell Biochemistry* 1995;22:1–10.

Martinez, M. E., et al. "Calcium, vitamin D and the occurrence of colorectal cancer among women." *Journal of the National Cancer Institute* 1996; 88:1375–1382.

Prasad, J. S. "Effect of vitamin E supplementation on leukocyte function." *American Journal of Clinical Nutrition* 1980;33:606–608.

Romney, S., et al. "Plasma vitamin C and uterine cervical dysplasia." *American Journal of Obstetrics and Gynecology* 1985;151:978–980.

Schiffman, M. H. "Diet and faecal genotoxicity." *Cancer Survey* 1987;6:653–672.

Shklar, G., et al. "Regression by vitamin E of experimental oral cancer." *Journal of the National Cancer Institute* 1987;78:987–992.

Tanaka, J., et al. "Vitamin E and immune response." *Immunology* 1979;38:727.

Thomas, M. K., et al. "The need for more vitamin D." *The New England Journal of Medicine* 1998;338:777–783, 828–829.

Wassertheil-Smoller, S., et al. "Dietary vitamin C and uterine cervical dysplasia." *American Journal of Epidemiology* 1981;114:714–724.

Zheng, W., et al. "Retinol, antioxidant vitamins, and cancers of the upper digestive tract in a prospective cohort study of postmenopausal women." *American Journal of Epidemiology* 1995;142:955–960.

CHAPTER 16

Alberts, D., et al. "Randomized, double-blind, placebo-controlled study of the effect of wheat bran fiber and calcium on fecal bile acids in patients with resected adenomatous colon polyps." *Journal of the National Cancer Institute* 1996;88:81–91.

Blot, W., Li, J. Y., et al. "Nutrition Intervention Trials in Linxian, China . . .", *Journal of the National Cancer Institute,* 1993, Vol. 85, No. 18, pp. 1483–1492.

Bostick, R., et al. "Calcium and colorectal epithelial cell proliferation in sporadic adenoma patients: a randomized, double-blinded, placebo-controlled clinical trial." *Journal of the National Cancer Institute* 1995;87:1307–1315.

Clark, L., et al. "Selenium in skin cancer patients." *Journal of the American Medical Association* 1996;276:1957–1963.

Duris, L., et al. "Calcium chemoprevention in colorectal cancer." *Hepatogastroenterology* 1996;43:152–154.

Habib, F. K. et al. "Metal–androgen interrelationships in carcinoma and hyperplasia of the human prostate." *Journal of Endocrinology* 1976;71:133–141.

Poo, J., et al. "Diagnostic value of the copper/zinc ratio in digestive cancer: a case-control study." *Archives of Medical Research* 1997;28:259–263.

Yu, S. Y., et al. "Regional variation of cancer mortality incidence and its relation to selenium levels in China." *Biological Trace Element Research* 1985;7:21–29.

Yu, S. Y., et al. "A preliminary report on the intervention trials of primary liver cancer in high-risk populations with nutritional supplementation of selenium in China." *Biological Trace Element Research* 1991;29:289–294.

CHAPTER 17

American Journal of Epidemiology 1994;139(1):1–

Ernst, E. "Can Allium vegetables prevent cancer?" *Phytomedicine* 1997; 4:79–83.

Hatono, S., et al. "Chemopreventive effect of S-allylcysteine and its relationship to the detoxification enzyme glutathione-S-transferase." *Carcinogenesis* 1996;17:1041–1044.

Li, G., et al. "Anti-proliferative effects of garlic constituents in cultured human breast cancer cells." *Oncology Reports* 1995;2:787–791.

Milner, J., Liu, J. "Prevention of 7, 12-dimethylbenz[a]abthracene induced mammary tumors by dietary garlic power supplementation." In: *Abstracts of the First World Congress on the Health Significance of Garlic and Garlic Constituents.* 1990:25.

Pinto, J., et al. "Garlic constituents modify expression of biomarkers for human prostatic carcinoma cells." *FASEB Journal* 1997;11:A439–A441.

Zylicz, Z., Hofs, H. P., Wagener, D. J. T., "Potentiation of cisplatin antitumor activity on L1210 leukemia s.c. by sparsomycin and three of its analagues." *Cancer Letters* 47:153–158.

CHAPTER 18

Adlercreutz, H., et al. "Inhibition of human aromatase by mammalian lignans and isoflavonoid phytoestrogens." *Journal of Steroid Biochemistry and Molecular Biology* 1993;44:147–153.

Bianchi-Salvadori, B., Vesely, R. "Lactic acid bacteria (LAB) and intestinal microflora." *Microecology and Therapy* 1995;25:247–255.

"Biotherapeutic agents: past, present and future." *Microecology Therapeutics* 1995;23:46–73.

D'Argenio, G., et al. "Butyrate enemas in experimental colitis and protection against large bowel cancer in a rat model." 1996;110:1727–1734.

De Stefani, E., et al. "Dietary fiber and risk of breast cancer. A case-control study in Uruguay." *Nutrition and Cancer* 1997;28:14–19.

Guerin-Danan, C., et al. "Milk fermented with yogurt cultures and *Lactobacillus casei* compared with yogurt and gelled milk: influence on intestinal microflora in healthy infants." *American Journal of Clinical Nutrition* 1998;67:111–117.

Kaaks, R., et al. "Dietary fiber and colon cancer." *Pathologie Biologie* 1994;42:1091–1092.

Kanazawa, K., et al. "Factors influencing the development of sigmoid colon cancer. Bacteriologic and biochemical studies." *Cancer* 1996;77(supplement):1701–1706.

Klein, S., et al. "Advances in nutrition and gastroenterology: summary of the 1997 A.S.P.E.N.

Pienta, K. J., et al. "Inhibition of spontaneous metastasis in a rat prostate cancer model by oral administration of modified citrus pectin." *Journal of the National Cancer Institute* 1995;87:348–353.

Platt, D., Raz A. "Modulation of the lung colonization of B16-F1 melanoma cells by citrus pectin." *Journal of the National Cancer Institute* 1992;84:438–442.

Rolfe, R. "Probiotics: prospects for use in *Clostridium difficile*–associated intestinal disease." Department of Microbiology and Immunology, School of Medicine, Texas University Health Science Center, 1996:47–66.

Stoll, B. A., et al. "Can supplementary dietary fiber suppress breast cancer growth?" *British Journal of Cancer* 1996;73:557–559.

Wang, C., et al. "Lignans and flavonoids inhibit aromatase enzyme in human preadipocytes." *Journal of Steroid Biochemistry and Molecular Biology* 1994;50:205–212.

Zoppi, G. "Probiotics and prebiotics in the treatment of infections due to vancomycin-dependent *Enterococcus faecalis* and of imbalance of the intestinal ecosystem (dysbiosis)." *Acta Paediatrics* 1997;86:1148–1150.

CHAPTER 19

Jankun, J., et al. "Why drinking green tea could prevent cancer." *Nature* 1997;387:501.

Komori, A., et al. "Anticarcinogenic activity of green tea polyphenols." *Japanese Journal of Clinical Oncology* 1993;23:186–90.

Kono, S., et al. "A case-control study of gastric cancer and diet in northern Kyushu, Japan." *Japanese Journal of Cancer Research* (Gann) 1988;79:1067–1074.

Nakachi, K., et al. "Epidemiological evidences for prevention of cancer and cardiovascular disease by drinking green tea." In Osawa, T. (ed): *Proceedings of International Conference on Food Factors—Chemistry and Cancer Prevention*. Tokyo: Springer-Verlag, 1997.

Oguin, I., et al. *Japanese Journal of Nutrition* 1989:47:93–102.

Satake, et al. Unpublished observations, 1996; see Fujiki, H., et al. "Japanese green tea as a cancer preventive in humans." *Nutrition Reviews* 1996;54:569.

Shimamura, T. "Inhibition of influenza virus infection by tea polyphenols." In Ho, Osawa, Huang, Rosen (eds): *Food Phytochemicals for Cancer Prevention II*. American Chemical Society, 1994:

Xu, Y., et al. "Inhibition of tobacco-specific nitrosamine-induced lung tumorigenesis in A/J mice by green tea and its major polyphenols as antioxidants." *Cancer Research* 1992; 52:3875–3879.

Yamane, T., et al. "Inhibition of N-methyl-N'-nitro-N-nitrosoguanidine–induced carcinogenesis by (-)-epigallocatechin gallate in the rat glandular stomach." *Cancer Research* 1995;55:2081–2084.

Yoshizawa, S., et al. "Penta-0-galloyl-B-D-glucose and (-)-epigallocatechin gallate." In Huang, M. T., Ho C. T., Lee C. Y. (eds): *Phenolic Compounds in Food and Their Effects on Health II.* Washington, D.C.: American Chemical Society, 1991:316–325.

Yu, T. G., et al. "Reduced risk of esophageal cancer associated with green tea consumption." *Journal of the National Cancer Institute* 1994;86:855–858.

Zheng, W., et al. "Tea consumption and cancer incidence in a prospective cohort study of postmenopausal women." *American Journal of Epidemiology* 1996;144:175–182.

CHAPTER 20

Cohen, S., Rabin, B. S. "Psychologic stress, immunity, and cancer." *Journal of the National Cancer Institute* 1998;90:3–4.

APPENDIX III

Ahn, D., et al. "The effects of dietary ellagic acid on rat hepatic and esophageal mucosal cytochrome P450 and Phase 2 enzymes." *Carcinogenesis* 1996; 17:821–828.

Barch, D., et al. "Structure–function relationships of the dietary anticarcinogen ellagic acid." *Carcinogenesis* 1996;17:265–269.

Hirose, Y., et al. "Chemoprevention of urinary bladder carcinogenesis by the natural phenolic compound protocatechuic acid in rats." *Carcinogenesis* 1995;16:2337–2342.

Hoffman, R., et al. "Potent inhibition of breast cancer cell lines by the isoflanonoid klevitone: comparison with genesteine." *Biochemical and Biophysical Research Communications* 1995;211:600–606.

Ip, C., et al. "Multiple mechanisms of conjugated linoleic acid (CLA) in mammary cancer prevention [meeting abstract]." *Proceedings of the Annual Meeting of the American Association of Cancer Researchers* 1996;37:A1905.

Loarca-Pina, G., et al. "Antimutagencity of ellagic acid against aflatoxin B: in the salmonella microsuspension assay." *Mutation Research* 1996;360:15–21.

Miller, C., et al. "Modulation of the mutagenicity and metabolism of the tobacco-specific nitrosamine 4-(methylnitrosamino)-1-(3-pyridyl)-1-butanone (NNK) by phenolic compounds." *Mutation Research* 1996; 368:221–233.

Ohnishi, M., et al. "Inhibitory effects of dietary protocatechuic acid and costunolide on 7,12-dimethylbenz(a)anthracene–induced hamster cheek pouch carcinogenesis." *Japanese Journal of Cancer Research* 1997;88:111–119.

Okuzumi, J., et al. "Inhibitory effects of fucoxanthin, a natural carotenoid on

N-ethyl-*N*-nitrosoguanidine–induced mouse duodenal carcinogenesis." *Cancer Letters* 1993;68:159–168.

Stoner, G., Morse, M. "Isothiocyanates and plant polyphenols as inhibitors of lung and esophageal cancer." *Cancer Letters* 1997;114:113–119.

Tanaka, T., et al. "Chemoprevention of diethylnitrosamine-induced hepatocarcinogenesis by a simple phenolic acid protocatechuic acid in rats." *Cancer Research* 1993;53:2775–2779.

Tanaka, T., et al. "Chemoprevention of colon carcinogenesis by the natural product of a simple phenolic compound protocatechuic acid: suppressing effects on tumor development and biomarkers expression of colon tumorigenesis." *Cancer Research* 1993;53:3908–3913.

Tanaka, T., et al. "Chemoprevention of digestive organs carcinogenesis by the natural product protocatechuic acid." *Cancer* 1995;75(supplement):1433–1439.

Thresiamma, K., et al. "Protective effect of curcumin, ellagic acid and bixin on radiation-induced toxicity." *Indian Journal of Experimental Biology* 1996; 34:845–847.

Thresiamma, K., Kuttan, R. "Inhibition of liver fibrosis by ellagic acid." *Indian Journal of Experimental Biology* 1996;40:363–366.

Udeani, G., et al. "Deguelin: a natural product for chemoprevention [Meeting Abstract]." *Proceedings of the Annual Meeting of the American Association of Cancer Researchers* 1996;37:A1905.

APPENDIX IV

Giovannucci, E., et al. "Physical activity, obesity and risk for colon cancer and adenoma in men." *Annals of Internal Medicine* 1995;122:327–334.

Mittendorf, R., et al. "Strenuous physical activity in young adulthood and risk of breast cancer (United States)." *Cancer Causes and Control* 1995; 6:347–353.

APPENDIX VI

Adachi, K., Nanba, H., et al. Potentiation of Host Mediated Antitumor Activity in Mice by Beta-glucan obtained from Maitake. Chem. Pharm. Bull. 35 (1) 262–270 1987.

Bougnoux, P., et al. Alpha-linolenic acid content of adipose breast tissue: A host determinant of early metastasis in breast cancer. *British Journal of Cancer* 1994; 70:330–334.

Brohult, A., Brohult, J., et al. Regression of Tumor Growth After Administration of Alkoxyglycerols. *Acta Obstetrics and Gynecology Scandanavia* 57:79–83. 1978.

Chinery, R., Brockman, J., et. al. Nature Medicine Vol. 3, Noll, Nov. 1997 p. 1233–1241.

Folkers, Karl., Biochemical and Biophysical Research Communications April 15, 1995; 192: 241–5.

Lamin, D., Riggs, D., Shriver, J., et al. Megadose vitamins in bladder cancer: a double-blind clinical trial. *J. Urol* 1994; 151: 21–26.

Lamm, DL., et al. *Cancer* 1997, 79: 1987–1994.

Levy, J., Karas, M., et al. Lycopene the major tomato carotenoid, delays cell cycle in breast, lung and endometrial cancer cells. Anticancer Research (1995) 15 (5A):1655.

Lockwood, K., Biochemical and Biophysical Research Communications July 6, 1995; 212:171–177.

Lockwood, K., Biochemical and Biophysical Research Communications March 30, 1994; 199:1504–8.

Mathew, B., Sankaranarayanan, R., et al. Evaluation of chemoprevention of oral cancer with Spirulena. *Nutrition and Cancer* (1995) 24(2): 197–202.

McNamee, D., Limone trial in cancer, The Lancet, Vol. 342, Sept. 25, 1993, p. 801.

Monti, E., Sinha, BK. Antiproliferative effect of genistein and adriamycin against human breast cancer cell lines. *Anti cancer Research* 1994, 14 (3A) p. 1221–6.

Sharoni, Y., Danilenko, M., et al. Lycopene inhibits cell proliferation in cancer cells. Anticancer Research (1995) 15 (5A): 1654–5.

Shklar, G.J., et al. *European Journal of Cancer* 1996; 32B: 114–9.

Stark, MJ., Burke, YD., et al. Chemotherapy of K-ras-transformed pancreatic carcinomas with perillyl alcohol, Proc. Annu. Meet.Am.Assoc. Cancer Research (1995)36: A2557.

Stark, MJ., Burke, YD., McKinzie, JH., et al. Chemotherapy of pancreatic cancer with the monoterpene perillyl alcohol. *Cancer Letter* 1995, 96 (1):15–21.

Stayrook, KR., McKinzie, JH. Induction of apoptesis by perillyl alcohol in pancreatic adenocarcinoma. *Carcinogenesis* 1997 18(8): 1655–8.

Tan, B. Antitumor Effects of Palm Tocotrienols in HRS-J Hairless Female Mice. Nutrition Research 1992: Vol. 12, Suppl. 1 p. 163–173.

Tiwari, R.K., et al., J. Natl. Cancer Institute. 1994 Vol. 86 No. 2 p. 126–131.

Index

309